"If grief is the language of love, this unflinching book shows us how to love a little deeper."
— Kate Bowler, author of *Everything Happens for a Reason (and Other Lies I've Loved)*

"In this disarmingly forthright and often funny book, Dana Trent reminds her readers that we're all terminal, and we'll all ride the grief train sooner or later—so why not start the conversation now? Her ability to convey what she has learned as a hospital chaplain, a daughter, and a teacher grounds every page in the real world, making it impossible to resist her invitation to begin thinking about The End in a lifegiving way."
— Barbara Brown Taylor, author of *An Altar in the World*

"We aren't very good at talking about death. Thankfully we have people like Dana to walk with us. Her writing here is approachable and honest, and her compassion overflows as she leads us into the difficult but necessary places. *Dessert First* is both a deeply moving and incredibly practical guide for dying (and living) well. It's essential reading for the mortals among us."
— John Pavlovitz, author of *A Bigger Table and Hope and Other Superpowers*

"*Dessert First* really helped me. It helped me prepare for the deaths of people I love. It helped me prepare for my own death. Don't worry: it isn't a book written by Miss Morbidity. Dana Trent is funny and professional and human, exactly the kind of person you want to help you face life's one actual certainty."
— Brian D. McLaren, author/activist

"*Dessert First* is a delicious treat—nourishing and enjoyable. A timely reminder not to neglect the things that matter most. Practical, truthful, needed."
— Philip Gulley, author of *If the Church Were Christian*

"What is a good death? How does one prepare? Dana Trent's *Dessert First* is a complete book. It is filled with practical wisdom gleaned from religious reflection and practical experience as an end-of-life chaplain. She has somehow transformed that experience into a joyful assessment of life and preparation for its end. Trent's wisdom comes in narrative form, which adds to the accessibility and, dare I say, enjoyment of this thoughtful book. It deserves many readers."

— Richard Lischer, Duke Divinity School, author of *Stations of the Heart: Parting with a Son*

"There is great freedom in accepting the reality of death. There is even joy. And possibly a great deal of humor. It is all here in *Dessert First*, a book about death that adds up to the fullness of life implied by the title. Dig in."

— Erin Wathen, author of *Resist and Persist: Faith and the Fight For Equality,* and Patheos blog *Irreverin*

dessert first

Preparing for Death while Savoring Life

J. Dana Trent

chalice
press

Saint Louis, Missouri

An imprint of Christian Board of Publication

Cover design: Jennifer Pavlovitz

ChalicePress.com

Print ISBN: 9780827206694
EPUB: 9780827206700   EPDF: 9780827206717

Contents

For Ron, with gratitude for all you did for Mom—and me.

Introduction:
We're All Terminal

*"You would know the secret of death. But how shall you find
it unless you seek it in the heart of life?"*
—Khalil Gibran, *"On Death,"* The Prophet

*"A book telling people how much I hurt would not do any
good. This had to be a book that would affirm life."*
—Harold Kushner, When Bad Things Happen
to Good People

"Is it a regional?" Mom used to ask.

Whenever I traveled by plane, she'd inquire as to an aircraft's size. If it held 100 passengers or less, her anxiety unfurled into a rant on the dangers of "puddle jumpers." This, coming from a woman who, as an infant, was flown in her father's two-passenger Cessna across state lines so that my grandmother could change her diaper.

But at the beginning of what became a turbulent regional ride from Atlanta from Birmingham, my mother's ever-present dis-ease with small planes rang true. Though Mom had died six months prior, as with most close mother-daughter relationships, her advice still haunted me.

The airline showed its innocuous emergency procedures video to us, a medium-sized congregation of unsuspecting passengers. We watched on headrest screens as earnest, cheerful employees parsed disaster protocol with far too much enthusiasm. Speaking from an array of skin colors, accents, body shapes, and sizes, they provided requisite information so that, should we plummet to our death mid-flight, *everyone* would do so *safely*.

In pressed navy uniforms and professionally whitened teeth, attendants demonstrated oxygen masks, signaled manicured hands toward floor-level exit lighting, and modeled inflatable life vests. The message was clear: *We're going to die in a way that meets federal aviation requirements.*

It was the first puddle jumper I'd taken since my mother died. This time, there had been no call to inquire, "Is it a regional?" I was 36 and mid-grief, facing the fact that I'd lived long enough to lose both parents, and beginning to wrestle with the idea that I was closer to the end of life than its beginning.

Why do these safety assurances, shown in every flight, every day, speak nothing of actual death? I wondered. *Why are we in such denial about our sure end? Why not tell us something useful during these plane didactics, such as what to say to our loved ones should we get the chance, rituals to keep from losing our minds mid-downward spiral, or prayers invoking the benevolence of whoever holds the keys to our (hopefully) glorious destination?*

My brother Ron, my mom, and I had seen the film *Sully* together. Mom had *loved* Tom Hanks's portrayal—but had also known there was only one *real* Captain Sullenberger.

And he was now retired. The once-in-a-million aircraft survival story had already been used up on the Hudson River.

Mom was now gone, but her disdain for "puddle jumpers" still echoed in my memory. Listening to the video of the flight attendant spiel, I wished that I were told something more true, more helpful, perhaps along these lines:

"In the event of a plane emergency, we *will* die. At that time, stuff yourself with as many of those delicious cookies or pretzels you want and place your oxygen mask on if it makes you feel better. But don't waste time fumbling for those damn water wings known as your seat cushion. Forget the exits; instead, review the multifaith rituals card we've placed in your seat pocket. Atheist? No worries. Breathe deeply anyway. Faith or no faith, take a second to switch off airplane mode and use whatever signal we have to text, call, or Facetime anyone you'd like. Hold hands with the passenger next to you; there's no time like the present to make new friends. As we make our final descent (literally), here are three useful ways to position your body to *ensure* you'll die on impact. No prolonged suffering on our watch! Thank you for choosing our airline."

"We're all terminal," I'd heard author Kate Bowler say in a lecture I attended six months after Mom died. "Some of us just have more information." I'd begun to heed *both* their insights: I *was* terminal—we all are—and I *could* die anytime—even in this metal tube 30,000 feet above the Southeast.

Long ago, I'd done research on the cause for Mom's anxiety: was there *real* danger in flying? Yes, at different points of the process. The likelihood of flight trouble is exponentially higher during taxi, right when they play that stupid safety video or perform the Gospel reenactment of "Federal Safety Regulations Require..." Danger also spikes during takeoff and landing.

On this trip, instead of studying the safety placard as instructed, I blared George Harrison's "My Sweet Lord" loudly in my ear buds and recited prayers to the beat. I thought of Mom. If this regional was going to seal my fate, so be it. Mom would welcome me at the pearly gates, while my earthly loved ones have their marching orders: comfort my husband, Fred, in his grief; and, make sure people laugh at my funeral.

I was under no delusions that this particular in-flight ritual kept me safer than the emergency management choreography. But when we finally parked and they turned off the fasten seatbelt sign, I thought: *Mom, it wasn't my time—yet.*

But one day—just like Kate Bowler and Mom cautioned, it will be. No oxygen mask, water wings, or hideous life jacket is going to keep me alive forever. My take on the ridiculous airplane video is that it's a metaphor for life: we can put all the life-prolonging safety measures we want in place—diet, exercise, expeditions to the "fountain of youth"—but, one day, we *will die.*

If I began the flight—or life—with the end in mind, I might *begin* to consider what *really* matters now—and what *will* matter in those last moments, hours, days, weeks, months, or years.

Why not be forthcoming about my—and our—shared fate? Certainly, no one wants to hang out with Miss Morbidity 24/7, but both of my mentors were right: Why not acknowledge the actual *terminal* nature of life? Why not embrace *some* time during taxi, take-off, and landing for a quick life review? Why not do a gratitude check of all the people who've loved and tolerated us? What might we then do or say to our loved ones should we arrive safely at the gate? Or, God forbid, should something go wrong, why not skip the oxygen mask and spend our remaining moments meaning-making?

"I'm boarding," I would always say as I was about to depart from the airport *terminal* (a term my mother considered as a metaphor for a stroll toward the grave). Like clockwork, Mom would always ask: "Is it a regional?" Followed by, "I hate those puddle jumpers," as if I'd never heard her tirade before. But she always followed the old standard by saying, "I'll start praying."

That, as it turned out, was actually useful.

The Death Chaplain

When I was 25, I spent a year gathering information about death without really meaning to. I was a freshly minted Duke Divinity School graduate and ordained Baptist minister beginning a hospital chaplaincy program. By chance (or perhaps not), I was assigned to serve patients at the end of their lives.

I became known as "The Death Chaplain." It was an unexpected call to an alternative universe—one in which, just inside the hospital doors, nearly all my patients were living the worst—and sometimes last—days of their lives. In that space, at 25, I learned what "terminal" truly meant. I saw it stamped vividly on cancer diagnoses, chronic disease, accidents, assaults, suicide—and even on births. As the death chaplain to these patients and their families, I immediately stepped into a world of endings I knew nothing about. All year, I learned essential lessons about facing the most challenging aspect of our lives: our dying.

Looking back, it's clear I began my chaplaincy year as a greenhorn, even though I *thought* I was a know-it-all graduate from a prestigious university seminary, fully trained in theology. I *did* know orthodoxy and scripture, and could read ancient manuscripts in their original languages of Hebrew and Greek. But no matter how many degrees I held, how many books I read, I still hadn't learned the single most important truth of life: we will die.

It the world of hospitals, death is a natural part of life. My mother and brother—a nurse and doctor respectively, had *lived* in this world. Neither of them skipped a beat over blood, guts, vomit, mangled limbs, diseases, or broken bodies. In their eyes, illness—and death—were a part of *life*. The two bravely showed up for the sick and accepted the facts. "It's just a body," they'd say, when I'd balk over some medical horror they shared.

But outside those concrete hospital walls, for a naïve humanities student such as myself (and many others), this ugly side of the fragility of these bodies is glossed over—forgotten or hidden under a shiny veneer of picture-perfect social media accounts and digitally enhanced Christmas card portraits.

Though the death rate is 100 percent, there is something about being terminal that *shocks* us. Maybe it's that we spend our entire lives trying to keep our bodies going, staying alive as best we can—from the poorest among us to the richest. We attempt to maintain bodies that, ultimately, cannot be sustained. We do not want to land in the Emergency Department, only to disappear from the future family portraits or status updates. We want to *live*.

But the greatest lesson my mother, brother, patients, their families, doctors, nurses, fellow chaplains, and dying loved ones taught me is that we *are* terminal. After sitting with over 200 dying people (not all at once), I learned to unwrap the gifts our finite bodies—and their deaths—offer us: reality, courage, and curiosity. I became a friend of "terminal," facing the fear in order to begin with the end in mind.

That is death's lesson: it teaches us how to live.

We're All Terminal

So, if we all die, why do we spend decades mastering skills and trades that change and disappear—while avoiding investing our time in that one certainty?

What if, instead, we gave some of that mastery to our biggest task, asking our biggest questions and embracing reality wholly? What if we opened ourselves to embrace the knowledge that we are *born dying*—would we *maybe* discover our truest and deepest *living* selves?

At a young age, even though I accepted biblical promises of my God's house of many mansions, I wore Doubting Thomas's robes. I longed for tangible evidence—blueprints and movie trailers—of what happens beyond this decades-long struggle of learning lessons too late. Heaven's architectural plans never arrived in my mailbox, but I did see glimpses of its mysticism in people's lives—and deaths.

In that early work as a Christian minister, theologian, and hospital chaplain, I learned the psychological and physiological processes of dying, the variations and nuances, from start to finish.

I also learned that modern medicine aids in a more comfortable, peaceful transition (for most of us working in hospital or hospice care). But what frightened me, and still squeezes the air from my chest, are the boundaries of our lifetimes and the obscurity of what comes after.

Before my chaplaincy, when I remembered that loved ones die and I will die, I used to melt into a puddle of tearful blubbering because I wouldn't *see, touch,* or *hear* from my loved ones again in this life. Until I began writing this book, I hadn't learned to befriend that normal, paralyzing fear; or the afterlife's mystery; or the deep, visceral grief we can feel when the door firmly shuts, and we are left behind to sort out its ending.

Because we are all in our various processes and understandings, this book is as much for me as it is for others. It is about learning to face death's reality in order to live our fullest lives—and ensuring that, when the time does arrive, we make it meaningful.

Death as a Meaningful Destination, Not a Dreaded Landmark

Perhaps the starting point means taking a step to embrace death as *real,* acknowledging it, and—heaven forbid—*talking* about it. How might we then learn practical skills, such as what to expect when loved ones die (and when we die), how to grieve, and what religion and spirituality can teach us about death and coping? How might we live with the end in mind?

When my mother was diagnosed with a sudden, terminal illness, both my brother and my husband were steadfast companions in sorting it all out. But what unspooled from there was a progression through the deep lessons I'd learned from being the death chaplain—understanding what it means to be "terminal," and understanding that everyone dies. These are the lessons I hope to share in this book, lessons that transform our journey, helping us to live fully awake in the now; lessons concerning:

1. what death is, why we avoid death, and how we can change our mentality about death;

2. what various religious and spiritual perspectives say about death and lightening the path; and

3. how we can plan for what the Catholic tradition calls a "good death"—employing rituals to help loved ones and ourselves in these transitions.

Finally, this book is meant to encourage each reader to do what may seem impossible in this moment: embrace death as a meaningful destination on the journey, rather than a dreaded landmark.

Laughter and Tears Are Not Mutually Exclusive

Don't worry, though, this book isn't a downer; it is not about hopelessness or helplessness. It's about empowering us to embrace reality and to give ourselves and our loved ones a sense of ownership—of acceptance—of our deaths, which subsequently increases our gratitude for our lives.

Yes, death can be devastating and sad. It can also be outright funny and curious and adventuresome; you'll meet stories across the spectrum in this book, and I hope you'll find yourself laughing out loud—even as you ask some of life's, and death's, biggest questions. Lean into that, too. This journey will be an uncovering and uplifting of what your soul already knows to be true so that your head and heart can catch up.

How to Use This Book

This book gives its reader space and tools to reflect on the hard questions we all ask. Alongside its narratives, *Dessert First* provides religious, spiritual, and practical resources on death and grief.

Depending on how you process living and grieving, the book offers different ways to respond and process that grief—be it journaling, talking, deeper reflection, or taking action.

Ultimately, this book is an invitation—to cease our unrealistic thinking that airline safety videos will ease the sting of the word *terminal.* My hope is that, over time, we'll all learn to embrace that inevitability: we are all terminal. I hope you'll let these chapters be your guide for preparing for that precious end—and living your best life until it arrives.

Whatever your situation—whether you feel devastatingly alone in your exploration and grief, or feel supported and comforted in it—my aim is to have the stories, reflections, and notes in this book help you on your journey. Know you are not alone in the grief, questions, wonderings, and life journeys. I invite you to consider this book your companion.

Chapter 1

Ashes to Ashes Road Tour

"[Y]ou are dust
and to dust you shall return."
—Genesis 3:19

"A mortal, born of woman, few of days and full of trouble,
comes up like a flower and withers,
flees like a shadow and does not last."
—Job 14:1–2, NRSV

Death is certain for all who take birth.
—Bhagavad Gita, Chapter Two, Text 27

"We'll buckle her in," undertaker Jake said, placing my mother's ashes in the passenger seat of my Honda Civic. "Just so she's safe," he added.

A slender, one-of-a-kind mortician, his effusive tenderness emerged from under a shoe polish mustache pasted under gaunt cheeks. His hair matched his suit, shiny and synthetic, as if he'd just emerged from the set of a CSI franchise.

Undertaker Jake offered his bereavement a bit too eagerly, embodying a modern paraphrase of Shakespeare's "The lady doth protest *too much.*" He was meek—until he wasn't. My brother, Ron, and my husband, Fred, considered this undertaker as two characters (after some experiences with him): gentle Jake, polite with customers in the *front* of the house, and gritty Jake—an expletive-ranting mortician hurling demands on behalf of the deceased in the back of the house.

We had evidence for our claim. After all, people get to know their funeral home associate when they've spent three hours cloistered in a conference room with him, surrounded by ceramic urns and "Remember Me" plaques.

After we shook hands and Jake offered his condolences, he plopped a thick folder of death paperwork on the table, and began. "What was your dear mother's *precious* name?" He whispered, pulling a pen from his suit pocket.

"Judith Wade Trent," we said.

"J-u-d-i-t-h," he spelled, *slowly,* as if he could no longer recall the speedy efficiency of his Yankee roots. In the 60 seconds it took to write six letters, I knew we'd be there all day.

"Date of birth?" he asked, barely audible.

Mom's membership in the Silent Generation elicited a monologue of military stories of war and woebegone days...

Later, he further interrupted his tortoise writing to interject a point of care:

"I treat your Mom like my own—if I see anything going on out back, well, aye—oh—aye—I'll let 'em have it."

What, precisely, would be going on "out back"? I didn't want to know.

We discovered his pristine mortuary ethics emerged from a complex family system. We also learned that he is "skinny enough" to do embalming.

"I can get back there where the other guys can't," he offered, proud. Was there no room at the mortuary to give a loved one a proper, roomy embalmment?

We passed on the embalming.

"They'll call you as she's going in," he said.

In, as *in* the cremation oven.

"Yes, please," I said, regretting my affirmative as soon as I uttered it.

Death, I had learned, churned the oddest sequence of events, feelings, and conversations. One minute, the three of us had been sitting at our dying mother's bedside, witnessing the thin space between here and eternity; then, in the next blink, we were spelling her name for a death certificate. One was profound; the other mundane. Months later, it occurred to me that this was death's constitution: the mystical transcendence of the human body, and the reality of being a human body. How could such meaningful, universal moments smack against such logistics? "Oh well, that's life in a beer barrel," Mom used to say whenever the sacred slammed into sensibility.

When we came to page five, Undertaker Jake asked if we'd like to see our mother. I nodded to Ron.

"Just to make sure she's dead," I whispered. "Seriously."

He accepted dutifully, because he's a wonderful big brother and a medical doctor.

"We'll get her all ready," Jake whispered, hand to his heart, disappearing like a vampire to the back of the house, where I imagined he rattled off orders to the team that they'd better make this lady look good, *or else.*

I drank Keurig cocoa while my brother and husband perused memorial merchandise and choked on coffin prices. We decided on a cardboard cremation box, an inexpensive sunset scattering box, and two silver urns the size of nesting dolls.

Jake re-emerged and led Ron to the dimly lit viewing room, where a screen separated them from Fred and me. Two minutes later, Ron returned, bringing a professional declaration of death.

"Dane, you gotta see her," he added. I wasn't certain. "She's beautiful," he assured. I followed him like I was four years old again, trusting my big brother not to lead me astray. We stood together and viewed our mother, stunning and angelic, laid peacefully in a temporary coffin, a euphoric sleep resting over her. Her cheeks were bursting with color, and her lips were pressed in her natural smile. The mauve prayer shawl a friend knitted hugged her chest, her arms draped gracefully over it. Fred's gift to her—a Hindu tulsi wood-beaded necklace—was wrapped around her right wrist; a Protestant glass-beaded prayer bracelet draped her left hand. They were symbols of the 48 hours of hospice vigil we'd just kept with her, representing Fred's Hindu and my own Christian traditions. Ron had been right: the three of us agreed that, throughout her life, we'd *never* seen her look so joyful as she did in death.

In that moment, I thought of taking a photo—a coffin selfie—but it seemed sacrilegious. I wish I had.

We gave Undertaker Jake our purchase choices, and he nodded. "Excellent," he added. Another hour of paperwork, and he walked us to the door, holding eye contact with effusive whispers of how well he'd take care of our dear, precious, lovely mother. The door closed behind us, and I felt someone should have yelled, "*Aaannnd…scene!*" so that Jake could unclip his tie, kick off his shoes, and say, "Thank God that's over. Tonight, we eat steak!"

The three of us indulged in a nice dinner. We ordered dessert *first* in mom's honor, because she never ate according to anyone's food pyramid but her own.

"How did you make sure Mom was dead?" I asked Ron, mouth full of chocolate pie.

"I used a technique we learned in med school," he said.

"What is it?" I asked. He then made a right fist, knuckles out, and pressed into Fred's sternum, and rubbed his hand up and down. My husband nearly spit out his bite in anguish.

"That hurts," Fred said. "I know," Ron replied. "Do me!" I commanded Fred, who mimicked Ron's trick. In the middle of the restaurant, the three of us took turns mimicking this painful gesture, called a "sternal rub," used by medical professionals to wake even those teetering on the edge of glory.

"Works every time," Ron added, and took another bite.

Life in a Beer Barrel

The weekend unfurled into the great tension of the first weeks of grief: deeply mourning a loss while enduring arrangements. I wanted to hide in a hole, but there were things to be done: paperwork and publicly honoring someone's life and legacy. It's like assembling IKEA furniture in a wind tunnel. Even as you grip the pieces to put together something useful, emotions swirl around you, hurling the parts in all directions. There was the busyness of phone calls, card reading, and service scheduling. Then, there were the moments that froze me in my tracks: *My God, she's not coming back. This is real.*

After we dropped my brother off at the airport and I bawled the entire car ride home, Fred determined we should watch *Gremlins* to give my mind a break. "It's a *Christmas* movie," he coaxed, hoping to offer me a two-hour reprieve from intermittent planning and sobbing. Midway through the movie, the crematorium called to say, "She's going in." The sobbing returned.

As Mom would have said, *"That's life in a beer barrel."*

The Tuesday after our afternoon with Jake, I walked back into the funeral home, alone. A front manager was swallowing his lunch, contorting his face from the satisfaction of a delicious sandwich to the soft sadness death industry workers can drop into quickly: "How *are* you?" He mumbled, finishing his bite.

I'd just finished teaching a college class, during which energetic adolescents made me forget that my mother was dead, and that death is even a thing amid such vibrant hopes. It took me a minute to remember why I was there, and why this guy was talking like someone had just died.

Never one to disappoint, Undertaker Jake appeared without prompting and greeted me with the same tenderness as before, which made me wonder how they know when to pause the funny cat videos they all must watch when no customers are in the building just to keep their sanity. He led me to the conference room for more paperwork. I signed the death certificate, and for her ashes and the metal tag that accompanied her body into the cremation oven. I held the tag in my hand, fixated. It was more surreal than her ashes, as if it held the energy of her last bodily existence. My eyes welled up, sad that Ron and Fred were not there with me, as they had been on Friday—pillars on which I could lean when these waves of reality struck.

"Let me carry these out to the car with you," Jake stepped in, gathering the death accoutrements containing what was left of my mother. We squinted in the bright summer sun, and he asked: "Where would you like her?" holding Mom's sunset scatter box in his arms like his very own infant.

"I was going to put her in the front seat with me," I stammered, because it only then occurred to me that the trunk was a bad idea.

"We can do that," he said. Then he opened my passenger door and *buckled Mom in.*

"There," he said, proudly patting her. "All safe."

He then placed the two silver urns in the cup holders. *Practical,* I noted. He walked me to the driver's side and offered his final condolences.

"You call if you need *anything*," he added.

I started my car and began driving my cremated, seat-belted mother home, but not before texting a friend a photo, getting an immediately reply: "You should take her through the drive through for a Frosty!"

Dessert *first*. She would have loved that.

"Ashes to Ashes" Road Tour

Mom's second seat-belted road trip came seven months later, when Fred and I buckled her in behind the driver's seat for a four-hour ride to South Carolina's low country.

This was where my mother had spent the happiest Augusts of her life. She stayed in a three-week timeshare she owned with her first husband, Dude—my brother's father.

Ron and my sister-in-law, Penny, had been anticipating our—and Mom's—arrival. After dinner that first night, we plotted how the four of us might clandestinely scatter a small portion of Mom's sunset box on what would have been her 78th birthday, two years shy of the octogenarian goal she'd set for herself.

Mom was ready for the tide to sweep her out to the Atlantic. But none of us were exactly prepared.

Ron, Penny, Fred, and I discussed logistics. We would scatter a small amount on the beach, and then take some of her remaining remains for a continued "holiday dispersal expedition" to Ohio, Indiana, California, and North Carolina—the four states she'd called home. The "Ashes to Ashes" Mom Tour would kick off here, with us, at her favorite South Carolina beach.

Her sealed sunset box sat atop the coffee table in the house my brother rented for spring break. We examined the small square perforation underneath the pull-off lid, pondering: *Should we break the seal now or later? What do we do once the slot is opened and the box has to continue to travel? Is duct tape an appropriate solution?* And: *How will we access the ashes from this tall box, which is only halfway full? Do we scoop her out? With what?* And most importantly: *Can we avoid arrest?*

Our two-hour deliberation concluded with our watching a YouTube video featuring a closing scene from *The Big Lebowski*. John Goodman ("Walter") and Jeff Bridges ("The Dude") are scattering the ashes of Steve Buschemi ("Donny"), who had been unceremoniously placed in a red Folgers coffee can with a purple lid. After Walter's elocution safari on Donny's character, the ashes are released upwind, only to cover "The Dude's" face.

"Let's hope that doesn't happen," Ron said.

The next morning, we awoke to heavy rain and 40 degrees: less-than-ideal conditions for Mom's "Ashes to Ashes" birthday debut. We waited for a break in the clouds, which arrived at two o'clock, and four well-educated but nervous adults carried our dead mother to a public access beach.

The parking lot was empty; we were puzzled, but relieved. Still, just in case we came upon a stranger, my sister-in-law—the best critical thinker among us asked: "Shouldn't we put her in *something?*"

"I've got her Trader Joe's bag," my brother answered.

"Perfect!" I added.

We carried Mom out to her favorite beach spot in her favorite grocery chain's bag, with the sun beaming brightly, but the water was choppy. At the end of the short boardwalk, we realized why no was there to catch us illegally scattering human remains.

The wind came in sheets, blowing sand in diagonal lines, like a Saharan storm. We hesitated, and the wind picked up. The only thing missing was *The Big Lebowski, Part II* film crew.

We were about to call it quits when Ron shouted above the howl, "Look!" A school of porpoises emerged in the water straight ahead. They were a mere 10 feet from the waves lapping the sand, playing as they darted in and out of the breakers. We took it as a sign—*our* sign—that the time was now.

We placed Mom on the sand carefully, against the blue sky and lush island trees, the cotton candy clouds framing her box, her life, and her beach. Photos were snapped to commemorate the moment; and, before the wind could blow her over, we surrounded her box in a semicircle to block the gales. Ron had chosen a beautiful poem to read. I hadn't given any "last words" two thoughts, which reminded me I was still waist deep in trauma and grief, mid-heartache that leaves no room for planning. I stumbled over unprepared words about what a pain in the ass she could be, but that she was *our* pain in the ass, and she'd been the one to bring the four of us together.

There, as the four of us stood on the Eastern shore, the universe seemed to widen. It was one of those mystical moments of meaning that you cannot describe, but makes you feel simultaneously finite *and* eternal. The thread that wove us together—our mother—would soon float out to the Atlantic.

After porpoises and eulogies, how does one *reverently* sprinkle into the ocean a portion of their Mom during a "small craft advisory," "gale force wind warning," and "seek shelter immediately" weather alert?

Mom would have said, "Very carefully."

The four of us didn't know we were releasing our mother in a verifiable wind storm until we returned to the house, where we learned that, according to the Weather Channel, we *should* have been filming *Big Lebowski, Part Deux: More Ashes*.

From tumbleweeding Kleenex to an ashes spill, to unceremoniously completing a *second* scattering when remains fell into the Trader Joe's bag, we inhaled brisk salty air and life lessons: check for weather advisories prior to tossing your dead parents into the sea. "Well," our mother would have said, hands on her hips, with an "I told you so" validation of her spending decades watching Jim Cantore rise to fame on the Weather Channel in a blue LL Bean parka. As with her recurring puddle-jumper PSA, *she* would have left a voicemail about any drizzle or breeze, let alone gale-force winds.

We stood on the shore as long as we could. The dolphins left, and she had, too. At the boardwalk, the winds calmed and we sat in swings, boasting at our accomplishment. When a large pinecone—the size of a cat's head—nearly knocked us out, we believed it to be Mom, who wanted some credit in the course of events…at least, for sending the porpoises.

This Is Not What It Looks Like

At the conclusion of spring break, we faced the task of dividing some of the remaining ashes for the continued road tour. Tupperware seemed appropriate, if not sacrosanct. Or, maybe glass bottles. We shopped the local surf joint for cheesy urn-ish containers, only to find small message-in-a-bottle vessels.

Fred and I bought our four with cork stoppers and set up shop. We had no funnels, no scoops, or even plastic spoons with which to transfer her ashes. Fred suggested we use aluminum foil. We made a makeshift funnel to transfer my dead mother from the sunset scatter box to four souvenir glass bottles labeled with "Pirates Map" and "My Place at the Beach."

When Ron came downstairs to check on our progress, Fred and I looked up from our focused sifting. "I promise we're not freebasing," I said. Ron nodded and went back upstairs. Since he'd been the one to check to ensure Mom was dead, he seemed relieved we'd take responsibility for divided ashes.

"All done," I said, as we poured the last bit into a glass skull-and-crossbones bottle. Fred smiled. You've found your life partner if someone willingly helps you transfer cremated remains into souvenir wine bottles for Barbies.

Chapter 2

The Gas Will Be Gone Soon

"To live in this world
You must be able
to do three things:
to love what is mortal;
to hold it...
and when the time comes...,
to let it go."
—Mary Oliver, *"In Blackwater Woods"*

"The gas will be gone soon," Mom whispered one morning in hospice. She didn't have much energy left. And what little life force remained was being slowly sifted through an hourglass none of us could overturn.

"Are you OK with that?" I asked.

"Yeah," she nodded, no strength to elaborate.

Mom had been in inpatient hospice for only four days before I began to feel parts of her "lift away" from us, like a heaven-bound balloon. She exhibited signs of shifting into what Celtic spirituality calls "thin spaces." These are the places of life at which the veil between this world and the next is translucent with mysticism, where the line between mortal and eternal blurs.

Most dying people experience thin spaces as odd and poignant messages conveyed from beyond earthly, finite life. "This place is a haunted house," Mom said one morning. Another time, she asked, "Did he leave?" And later, "Did you hear that dog?" I imagined the spiritual visitors she must have been receiving in those last days: her father and his dog, her mother, brother, sister, and former husbands. A few times, she even laughed in her sleep, and I wondered what stories they must have been telling, reassuring her what would lie beyond her dying body.

Ron, Fred, and I had been at her hospital and hospice bedside for two weeks. At age 77, she'd been admitted to the intensive care unit on a Tuesday evening with internal bleeding and diverticulitis with perforation, a very serious but treatable condition. She was an otherwise healthy older adult with no chronic diseases. She was lucid and capable. Ron, my doctor-brother, who also held her health-care power of attorney, helped her articulate and advocate for the level of hospital care she'd always wanted. "No knives," she'd told us both repeatedly. This declaration initially left green-scrub–clad surgeons baffled, even as they explained that her condition, without their scalpel, was terminal. To them, "the knife" was a simple life extender.

But the primary surgeon honored her request to be stabilized only. He and Ron prepared a plan of care: enough blood transfusions, saline, antibiotics, and pain meds to enjoy family visits for one last three-day weekend reunion, with goodbyes. She would then be transferred to a palliative care team who would organize her inpatient hospice admission. There, she'd receive ample pain, anxiety, and secretion medication to cope with her final days—when her body would become septic.

"Judy's Party," was what we called that weekend at the hospital. Flowers and gifts adorned her room. The grandchildren flew in; nieces and nephews came from far and wide. Mom's only living sister sat by her bedside. We shoved chair after chair into her room, and broke all visitation rules. Ron set up a speaker by her bedside and made a "Mom" playlist. Music was blared, stories shared, photoshoots performed, and contraband chocolate milkshakes snuck past the "NPO" (nothing by mouth!) sign taped to her door. She raved over the spoonfuls of chocolate goodness Ron fed her, and even danced to the "Freebird" guitar solo.

Our mom *loved* the busyness of hospitals; she'd worked in them for decades. It was the perfect setting for her party. Hospice was much harder for her. Family flew, or drove, home; visits slowed down and most days were quiet. Though we were alone a lot, I'm not certain that the reality of losing my mother ever hit visceral level. My body rushed with cortisol from the onset of her sudden illness; I felt the urge to remain stoic. I knew I couldn't facilitate "a good death" for Mom from puddles of tears. I put on my death chaplain hat and vowed to give her the best death possible. And I knew how to do it.

The Blue Room

Mom's favorite movie was *Out of Africa*. When I was in middle and high school, she played its soundtrack every morning, drank coffee, and read. The complexity of the story—its characters, disappointments, landscapes—enthralled her. She was enveloped by this fantasy world— where, at her best, Baroness Blixen was the woman my mother wanted to be: wealthy, brave, and compassionate.

At her hospice death bed, I played her worn *Out of Africa* CD on repeat. She'd perk up at the composition crescendos, telling me I was her "bestest buddy." Mom commented on what I wore, including the red James Taylor concert T-shirt, a holy relic from a show we had attended together. I tried to surround her with her favorite things and cherished memories. We taped up photos around the sky-blue room and read from her favorite books.

In between moments of rest, reading, short conversations, and music, I typed on my laptop. "I'm writing about you," I told her. "I'm writing about this journey with you." Hearing that, she smiled and laid her head back down on the pillow.

I had hoped to give Mom a "good death." But dying is hard. It wasn't the swift fairy tale death afforded to many of my intensive care unit patients during that chaplaincy year. Most of the 200 transitions I'd seen as the death chaplain were heavily sedated or comatose patients on total life support, who, when the medical technology was all withdrawn, departed from life swiftly and tenderly, without awareness of discomfort or the cognitive burden of two weeks of marching toward death. Back then, my primary job had been to be present and make the passage meaningful. I was to honor any religious, theological, or spiritual rituals they or their families wanted; ensure their dignity; and offer care and comfort for their loved ones and staff.

Mom's dying was different; there was no seamless withdrawal of breathing tubes and ventilators offered in tandem with doses of morphine that removed any feeling of suffocation. Mom had to endure the body's complex and reluctant shutdown process organ by organ, a process taking days, or even *weeks*.

There are times when I review those eight inpatient hospice days with regret: we had so much time with her—not mere minutes, the way it had been with my patients. Reflecting on the time, I ask myself what part of the journey I did not take with her. We could have had a lengthy life review—what might I have said, what should I have said, had I not been so tired and weary of making death more graced, painless for her? Six months after her death, I realized I hadn't even acknowledged so much that was basic and true to her situation, beginning with how hard it must have been for her to lose her life to pain, to immobility, to helplessness at the age of 77.

Years before Mom's death, a Hindu practitioner told me about her own experience of being with a loved one during end-of-life. She described it as the five senses leaving the body one at a time, and the dying person's consciousness slowly turning inward, growing more withdrawn and quiet. An oncology chaplain friend recounted the same experience with her own mother, and her realization that, though she too had wanted to talk endlessly with her mom about life and death, she realized that her mother simply hadn't had the energy to do so. It was only *after* the blue hospice room, when I recalled those words, that I tried to comfort myself with the fact that Mom was *not* up for constant chatting and engagement; she was turning inward to go home.

Sticky Notes

In the 1980s, Mom kept a blue sticky note pad on her desk that read, "From the Desk of God." On it was a cartoonish "old-man-looking" God with a lightning bolt striking from his robed arms. In those hospice days by her bedside, I felt like I needed a tap on the shoulder from God and one of those sticky notes.

Maybe the first one would have read, "Just be."

Or, perhaps, "It will all work out; don't worry about when or how. Only I know that. You've said and done all you need to. Now, just relish every moment together." I imagined the God-notes would have helped guide the time.

Instead, I was what Mom would have called, "anxious as a pole cat." Every minute was spent ensuring she was comfortable, not lonely or fearful during those eight days. I fretted over parts known and unknown: *Will we be able to adequately control her suffering as her body becomes septic? What if her body rallies and we get kicked out of hospice for being "too well"? What if she has to return to assisted living, only to enter the revolving door of hospital life for this condition that will, without surgery, ultimately, kill her? How long will we be here?*

It was a constant frenzy of push-pull, of life and death. Of pole-cattery and only little slivers of peace.

Another sticky note I would have wanted from God was a line Frank—a priest comforting author Kate Bowler after her Stage IV cancer diagnosis—had offered. "Don't skip to the end," he'd said.

The Labor

But the end *did* skip quickly forward. On day six, I worried and fretted 24/7. As her advocate and detective, I looked for symptoms of discomfort and clues of imminent death: urine output, color changes, skin that was cool to the touch—all indicators of her active dying; that she was in sepsis, a full-body infection resulting from the unrepaired intestine. I watched carefully for furrowed eyebrows and grimaces from the pain of sepsis—a terrible way to die, actually—and signs of her needing more comfort measures. Hospice increased her pain and anxiety meds when they were needed, while Fred, Ron, and I kept round-the-clock vigil, trying to be present with her in every hour, every breath. My work as the death chaplain had been exhausting because of its volume. Mom's death was exhausting because of its proximity. I was losing the very first part of me.

For the final 48 hours, she was *actively* dying. During that time, I recited revered soothing words to the music of *Out of Africa*. I read Mary Oliver poems, Psalm 23, and *The Prophet* by Khalil Gibran. A church deaconess brought lotion that filled the room with the scent of mint essential oil and helped us remember that human touch is important. Hospice continued to care for Mom's body with affection: bathing her, rubbing her with the lotion, cleaning her mouth with damp sponges, and braiding her long silver hair.

The last night she lived, Ron slept in the recliner across from her while Fred and I dozed on the pullout sofa beside her bed. We took shifts by her bed, held her hands, and rubbed her back. She hovered in the in-between stage our bodies must go through. But she wasn't ready just yet.

At one point, Ron and I surrounded her, on either side; he sat quietly, facing her and reading *The Wall Street Journal,* while I climbed into her bed and spooned her back. We each held her in our own loving ways, connecting with her remaining breaths as best we could.

She fell deeper into her sleep. In hospice, her vital signs were no longer measured by machines, so we used stethoscopes and visual cues. Ron's medical training taught him to decipher these well; I listened to her death rattle with hyper-alertness and watched her chest, neck, skin color, eyes, and brows, obsessed with intuiting if she needed more comfort measures by the signs her body showed us.

Thursday morning, at 7:00 a.m., we were relieved to see Katie, a nurse whom we'd had often before during our hospice stay. We all agreed Mom seemed "stable" in her dying, so Ron and Fred left hospice to move Mom's belongings from her assisted living apartment into storage.

At 11:30 a.m., Mom received more pain meds just before her next "turn." Our bodies, even if dying, must be moved every few hours; otherwise, blood pools, pressure sores can develop, and the tissue can become necrotic. In ICU, we had special pressure beds that inflated and deflated to mimic turns. But in these hospice beds turns were traditional; they helped with the airway secretions that cause the "death rattle," a troubling breathing sound that frightens the living. I hated these turns—but understood their utility. Past turns had elicited moans and eyes that looked scared and disoriented. Mom's level of consciousness during these mandatory movements shocked and upset me. Katie ensured that she would do her best to make this one less painful than the previous ones. They turned her on her left side, facing me. I could sit and talk with her easily.

After the turn, I sat on the pull-out couch and watched Mom breathe while a hospice volunteer wheeled in a tea cart with porcelain cups—the kind my Southern mother adored—and offered me a blueberry scone. I ate it bedside and chatted with Katie, who had shown us so much love and care. We talked about the spirituality and energy our loved ones emit as they leave us—

we had both seen *so many* people die. And Katie and I exchanged notes on that mystical, universal force that remains unseen: that spark from which we have all been crafted—the one you can *feel* as it leaves the body and the room.

Katie left to care for her other patients, and promised to check back in soon. I wandered over to the sink to "get dressed and act like I'm somebody," as my mother would have said. I started talking with her as I brushed my teeth, a habit that drove her crazy. Then, I walked back over to the couch to straighten the sea of blankets, telling her, "Mom, I'm straightening up." I told her what she probably already knew. She called me a biblical Martha at heart; tidying is my go-to coping mechanism. And I'd been doing this since she'd first been admitted to the hospital.

Hospital chaplaincy training taught me to *always* talk with the patient and tell them *exactly* what you are doing, all the time. You're on *their* turf—and the only control they have when they are conscious is to tell you *not* to do something. If they are unconscious, you *still* talk with them as if they may be awake and alert; medical research suggests that hearing is the last sense to leave as we die.

"Mom, everyone keeps telling me that maybe I should leave for a while," I said. "They remind me you may need some space—some privacy. You make not want to make...your *transition* with me here," I added, fluffing pillows.

I heard a loud, distinct gulp.

"Mom?"

I moved closer.

She breathed like a fish out of water—a final respiratory stage most of us will reach, should our deaths be slower than an instant. "Mom, did you hear me?" I asked, and pulled the chair up to her bed. This was a new breathing pattern for her—distinct from the sporadic Cheyne-Stokes, end-of-life, breathing pattern she'd had as we'd kept vigil.

I trusted my chaplain training when they insisted patients could hear me, and how a familiar voice might be muffled but comforting to the dying. What I hadn't trusted was Mom's higher level cognitive function. Because her respirations were now more sporadic, I imagined her brain's ability to process to be limited. I hadn't anticipated that Mom would *understand* what I'd said and be able to evaluate its meaning. But 30 minutes before with Katie and Melissa, she'd *opened* her dark brown eyes with a sense of knowing what was happening to her.

I sat down and held her hand.

"Did you hear me when I said I was going to leave?"

Her breathing changed again.

"You don't want me to leave?"

She gulped again. In that moment I understood two things: she was ready to go, and she wanted me there with her. For 48 hours we had kept vigil by her hospice bed, with endless prayers and scripture reading. We hung on to her every breath, wondering if it would be her last. She kept going until I was so tired and weary I'd almost given in, left the room, thinking she wasn't ready—or that she was, but wanted to go without me.

Then, taking both of her hands, I let her know I would stay: "I'm right here, Mom." One of her hands was draped with prayer beads and the other a tulsi necklace.

She gulped again—the body's signal that the very end was beginning. It was as if a labor was beginning.

"Mom," I spoke with the same tone she'd had with me when I was young and afraid and had to do something new. It had been this way for over three decades—our reliance on one another— the complex intertwining of a single mom and her only daughter; best friends and survivors who depended upon one another.

"We're going to do this together. I'm right here. We'll walk through it together... Concentrate on God; go *toward* God... The Lord is my Shepherd, the Lord is my Shepherd..."

When she was a little girl on her daddy's farm, she'd recite Psalm 23 when she walked the acreage by herself; it made her feel less alone, she said.

"The Lord is my Shepherd... God is that light you see and the love you feel... Don't struggle to stay back. We will be OK; you've given us all we need to survive. Focus on God; Jesus is there with open arms, ready for you. The Holy Spirit will guide you. I will miss you forever..."

She gulped and took another breath.

"Don't hesitate," I reminded her, encouraging her to focus only on God. I was *determined* that her last moments and thoughts would be focused on the faith she'd lived her entire life, the love we felt for her, her peaceful destination, and that we would be OK.

"The Lord is my Shepherd... The Lord is *your* Shepherd. I'm right here, it's OK to go..."

In her dying, I became her "doula." Through tears, I kept gently talking, and held her hands tightly, grateful she'd chosen me as a companion and this moment to travel from life to death.

Finally, her lips paled and her gasps silenced... She was gone. I looked at the clock: 12:26 p.m.

She had labored me into birth, and mothered me 36 years. And she'd given me the honor of helping her labor into the world beyond.

"The doctor said I labored beautifully," she'd told me each year when she recounted my birthday outside of Los Angeles. "You were born at 4:04 p.m., and I was sitting up in bed and eating supper by 5:00 p.m."

And so it was that I found myself alone at her bedside at the end of my earthly journey with her, the tables turned.

She had labored beautifully.

Gone

I pressed her bedside button; Katie and Melissa ran in.

"She's gone," I told them, and recounted the last minutes. They gasped and cried and left to file the official paperwork and record the time. I had a strange feeling of euphoria. The bubble of love and light, of feeling held and heard—of all your life's work and memories and loved ones wrapped in a delicate ether that cannot be seen nor contained. That's what it felt like for my mother's soul to shed its worn-out, septic body, and move into the afterlife. At first I didn't feel sadness—I felt as if I were floating.

My brother and Fred returned to her room a few minutes later with my cousin. I felt guilty that Ron wasn't there in those final moments with our mother, but realized that when a person is close to death, they often have a kind of unanticipated control, determining who needs to be there, who needs to *see* them transition, and those with whom they've left things peaceful and tidy. They also can determine if they need to labor alone.

For decades Mom would say, *conspiratorially,* "It's you and me against the world." In the end, it was still her and me; that's how she wanted it. That's how mothers and daughters sometimes are.

When the others arrived, my body shook as I recounted the unbelievable sense that she heard and understood me, and how her subsequent death labor had begun.

Postmortem

That floating feeling I had after Mom died—as if I'd just caught the Spirit at an old-fashioned tent revival—soon disappeared. It was strangely energetic, a relief from her suffering and mine. And yet, when I saw her cold, lifeless body—looking as if it were sleeping in its hospice bed—the loss hit me. My mother was gone forever.

Later that night, as I rode home from a "dessert-first" dinner with Ron and Fred, we rolled the windows down to listen to the late August sounds. It was the first evening of my life my mother wasn't alive. It was then that I realized she'd never hear another late summer nightfall—and that when I woke up the following morning, I'd live my first day ever without my Mom.

Lessons in Midwifery

Mom's death labor had been the culmination of 13 years of her own learning and living with death—professionally and personally. But *my* grief journey had now only begun.

Two months after Mom died, I shared dinner with a wise Hindu grandmother who asked for *specific* details about my mother's death. This genuine interest in the question shocked me—most people don't ask. It's a mistaken assumption that the bereaved do not want to recount their loved one's experience. In fact, many people tell stories of traumatic accidents over and over in the days and weeks following; they are trying to process them. But rarely is that space held for them, except by specialized chaplains, therapists, or empathetic family members. The bereaved have a particular need for folks to ask—or, better yet, to *remember* their loved ones and *say their names*. It keeps them *alive* for us.

This Hindu grandmother was an eager listener— empathetically eager to hear about Mom's death experience, and wanting to know my own perception and reception of it. When I finished recounting it all, without skipping a beat she declared: "You were her midwife. We all need midwives." Then she added: "In birth, *and* in death." She described how midwives keep us focused on the goal: the healthy birth of the child—or, in death, the realization of the "Ultimate Purpose," the "destination," however that looks for our religious, spiritual, or moral tradition. These midwives (whether they are recorded or not) are a part of the two most important pieces of paper we are assigned during our human experience: our birth certificates and our death certificates. "The dash"—as it's been poetically described—is what happens between. We need our midwives both at the beginning, *and* end—plus a slew of guides for the dash in between.

I hadn't realized it then, but I had been a "death doula" for all those patients and families that year at the hospital. I'd sat with them in that liminal space—the mystical time between life and death. My midwifery education began in that chaplaincy residency year after divinity school. That year of study and practice, of hours spent listening and sitting with patients as they took the mystical journey toward what lies beyond—helped prepare me for those 14 minutes on August 24, 2017, when my mother took her last breaths, with me right by her side.

Chapter 3

The Death Chaplain

*"This is my attempt to make sense of the period that
followed, weeks and then months that cut loose any fixed
idea I ever had about death, about illness, about probability
and luck, about good fortune and bad."*
—Joan Didion, The Year of Magical Thinking

The Death Chaplain

I walked into the hospital at age 25.

I was fresh from seminary, still six years from marriage, and living with Mom in the apartment we shared. Two months prior to my first day, we'd celebrated my acceptance into the chaplain residency program over quesadillas. She'd prepped and then driven me to the interview, and waited fervently for "all the details." It wasn't even an hour before they called to tell me I'd been accepted. Timing had worked in my favor. A confirmed candidate had dropped out, and, though I was a last-minute applicant, they needed to fill the slot quickly—even if it was with a fresh divinity school grad with no prior training in hospital chaplaincy.

Oh, what the hell! I imagine the interview committee must have thought. *Let's give this girl a shot.*

Mom and I lived that residency year *together*. She helped me decipher the way of hospitals: diagnoses and jargon. Ron—as a doctor—helped me understand the medical school educational nuances with which physicians can (or can't) handle life and difficult conversations with emotional patients and their loved ones.

It was a family affair; my mother, father, and brother were all health-care professionals. I had been the oddball: the creative dreamer/storyteller who majored in French and History—a pleasant but impractical education—and then went to seminary. My chaplaincy year was the year I finally understood the pull of their world—the excitement of deciphering symptoms and behaviors in order to solve mysteries and help the suffering, living in tandem with devastation when the offer of human help wasn't enough. It would also become the year in which I learned to understand human limits, fragility, and death.

Day one of my chaplaincy residency, my fellow chaplains enthusiastically declared their informed decisions regarding specialty chaplaincy areas they wanted to work in. I'd never even made hospital visits to parishioners before. Our CPE (Clinical Pastoral Education) supervisor laid out the unit options that could become our care specialties during the next year: Neurology and Psychiatry; Trauma and Surgery; Pediatrics; Cardiology; Oncology, and the Medicine Service.

I called Ron, panicking over my medical inexperience, my lack of hospital jargon. The five other chaplain residents had each had at least one unit (three months) of CPE training prior to being admitted, which qualified and equipped them to be fulltime chaplains on *any unit* in what was considered one of the most prestigious post-graduate level programs in hospital clinical pastoral care.

The Medicine Service sounded innocuous (wasn't it *all* medicine?), so I raised my hand to accept that one. Later, Father Truitt—the outgoing Medicine Service chaplain resident—cautioned me: this hospital's medicine service was far from mundane "medicine"; it included the Medicine Service Intensive Care Unit, or MICU, a floor whose deaths per capita far out-numbered any other in the hospital. The MICU was literally the last stop; if the MICU couldn't save you, *no one could.*

Everyone loved Father Truitt; he was an "all-American"-looking priest with an incredible bedside manner. He had been dubbed "the death chaplain," a moniker bequeathed to me, as

I succeeded him. I know I poorly filled his large Catholic shoes in my early weeks in training in CPE. Father Truitt offered wise caution: succeeding him as the death chaplain would force me to confront looming life questions most of us would rather avoid.

That forced confrontation would aid me in my role as a death doula for my mother many years later, but its beginnings were here, in one of the state's Level One Trauma Centers. As resident chaplain, I was responsible for one year of 8-to-5 day-shifts, plus 32 *additional* 24-hour, on-call, overnight shifts, during which I was to remain at the hospital. This meant that I assisted the MICU in caring for the majority of their patient deaths that year.

And because I had *absolutely no experience with death,* Father Truitt suggested I focus on only one goal that first month: *survival.* My chaplain supervisors supported me wholeheartedly, knowing I would quickly find out what death looked like, with the MICU offering me immersive experiential learning. They were veteran chaplains in the final decades of their careers, and they'd seen just about everything. They encouraged me to watch, witness, study, care, and observe the lived experience of death, dying, and dealing with grief's basic questions: *What happens when we begin to die? How do we care for those who are dying? What happens the moment we die? How do we care for the grieving? What happens within us as we self-reflect on caring for those who are dying, as well as their loved ones?*

The year would unfurl in deaths whose answers were never finite nor binary. Each death unfolded uniquely on its own, but with silken threads that wove a tapestry of understanding as to what we fundamentally want, need, and think when faced with life's end.

I would survive my residency year only because of Mom's endless capacity for listening, the secondhand celebrity magazines the hospital's library stocked in bulk, mindless episodes of *The Young and the Restless,* and my supportive chaplain colleagues.

I had assumed that anyone could do this death work. I was wrong.

But it suited me, and I soon learned why: the number one rule of chaplaincy—and ministry—is that you cannot sit with others in their pain and suffering unless you *know your own.* When I spent the first weeks of chaplain residency peeling back the layers of my own grief—losing grandparents and other loved ones at an early age—I began to learn best practices and care standards for those in their deepest emotional and physical pain.

Living among the Dead

It helped, too, that the MICU *needed* me nearly from day one. I lead with Enneagram Type 2 (the Helper) and ENFJ on the Myers-Briggs. To be useful, encouraging, and *needed* by others energizes me. The MICU was the perfect fit; they *needed* me to be present with patients and their families during the spiritual and mystical transition from this life to death. Once I realized what my work would look like, I felt as if God had been just waiting to show me this world.

As weeks passed, I grew eerily comfortable holding space and giving witness to patients' and families' pain, suffering, exhaustion, relief, and handling tough conversations with doctors—which often required fraught and seemingly impossible decisions. I discovered I worked best in crises spaces, sharing life with people having one of the worst—or at least "most defining"—days of their lives.

I think my CPE supervisor may have described my first semester best: "Dana took to chaplaincy in this setting as a morning glory takes to sunlight." Crisis *and* death *and* grief felt like home, even in the most exhausting circumstances.

I couldn't fill Father Truitt's shoes, so I cobbled together my own. One month in, I hit my stride, and embraced my identity as the death chaplain, even as it looked different from Father Truitt's chaplaincy.

By the year's end, I had been present for so many deaths that I learned to become absorbed in each patient's *entire* experience of death. My day-one focus of survival moved to wanting the people I cared for to feel seen, heard, and held. I learned to be comfortable with pain and mourning, and even silence. Within that, I learned self-reflection, too, understanding my own trauma and pain—which made me more empathetic in helping others hold theirs.

Living among the dead for a year changed everything.

The commonplace became catastrophic: *Is this my* last *bus ride home? Are these sniffles* just *a cold?*

It also became meaningful: *This could be my* last *meal with my mother, or my* final *sunset.*

Moving within the world as if I hadn't just spent all day caring for five dying people and watching them leave this life was impossible. Each day, MICU duties left an impression. The work also gave me an unquenchable hunger for life and meaning-making. And it made me lonely; I knew a secret no one else seemed to have discovered—or, at least, one they didn't want to talk about: we were *all* dying.

Chaplain or Satan? Satan or Chaplain?

With each new shift, there was a different pace and feeling in the hospital halls. During first shift, caffeinated colleagues buzzed back and forth through a main corridor with tall windows; the sun reminded you that you were still alive. During the second and third shifts, however, there was no sense of the balance of life and death, or daylight.

Chaplain on-calls—during which we worked 24 hours straight to cover *every* shift for the entire hospital—mirrored those zombie movies people told me about: Who's alive? And who's *really* dead? My mother worked second and third shift much of her nursing career. In emergency room and crisis work, she loved the fast-paced excitement of the "dark" hours. When she worked inpatient psychiatry, she appreciated the quiet of the medicated sleep of the otherwise psychotic people she served during their waking hours.

For chaplain residents, on-calls meant that, in addition to our regular daytime duties, we were responsible for *any* and *all* pastoral care needs in the entire hospital. Overnight shifts in a Level I Trauma Center were a siren call going out from the Statue of Liberty of sick people: "Give me your *most critical* patients in the state—your 90-percent burn victims, your fatal snake bites, your traumatic amputations, and your most disturbed mentally ill. Send these—I lift my lamp beside the Emergency Department sliding doors."

A one-week snapshot of on-call looked like this: four dying burn unit patients; three motorcycle accidents with amputated limbs in red biohazard bags; two suicide attempts—one by gunshot, the other via antifreeze; two brain stem herniations; two babies born premature without fully developed lungs; one meth lab explosion victim; and a schizophrenic *"pa-a-artridge in a pear tree."*

Patients came in droves throughout the night via ambulance or helicopter. My mother—still a night owl from those decades of overnight shifts—would phone me when she heard the chopper fly over our apartment, which was just two miles from the hospital: "You've got another one coming in," she'd say, just as the page came through on the old-fashioned trauma beeper.

On-call had its own kind of exhaustion in MICU. In between responding to the hospital's chaos, I served my own assigned patients and their families. Nights were dotted with cat naps and *People* magazine, heavy with loneliness amid emergency room deaths and family conferences. When I was finally released at noon after a 28-hour hospital shift, I emerged into the day stunned by the bright, strange world of traffic jams and people in a hurry—a world that went on as if no one were dying.

I began to develop coping mechanisms for those nights when the building was *too* quiet, *too* dark—the cling of death too real. Between emergency room prayers, delivering terrible news to families, and comforting the dying, I curled up in the twin bed of our on-call room to binge-watch reality TV and celebrity gossip—a glittery reminder that someone out there was still living...until my three pagers beeped again.

The MICU loved it when I was on-call, as I was "their person." The continuity from day shift to night shift made them and the patients and families feel more secure, so they didn't hesitate to page. The Emergency Department was also a frequent user of night chaplains. The ED was far more chaotic than MICU, which prided itself on calm staff and peaceful ambiance—to aid in "good deaths." In contrast, the ED staff kept their sanity with rambunctious and raucous chatter with their "walkie-talkies" (patients who are conscious and can walk and talk) at 3 a.m., or *anytime*. You *never* knew who or what would come into the ED at night—from diabetic grandmas to meth lab trailer fire victims. The ED also *loved* having chaplains on site; we kept the agitated "walkie-talkies" comforted and any pestering, anxious families out of the staff's way.

I responded to Level I trauma calls occurring after midnight in my all-black Fila tracksuit that doubled as pajamas. On occasion, the dark fabric against my pale skin seemed to have the unintentional consequence of creating the impression in the minds of tweaked-out patients that the Grim Reaper had arrived—only, she'd left her scythe at home. (Perhaps I should have rethought my attire.)

One time, when I was asked to update a patient's wife on his condition following a dirt bike accident, I frightened "Mrs. Dirtbike," who—when she saw my black track suit and "Chaplain" badge—screamed: "Oh my God, oh my God! My God! He's dead, ain't he? My Johnny is day-ed!"

"No ma'am—Johnny's *not* dead; he's going to be OK," I said, because Johnny was in fact not *anywhere* close to death.

"I need a cigarette!" she screeched, turning away from me and running for the ED exit.

"Go have a cigarette, come back, and we can talk," I called after her.

While I waited, the ED staff asked me to pray with a pending psychiatry inpatient admission lying on a gurney in the hall.

"Chaplain!" The red-headed, middle-aged woman reached out for me as soon as I approached.

"Oh, chaplain," she said, crying.

"Tell me how you're feeling tonight," I said, trying to open a "door" to gather clues as to how to care for her.

"Pray for me, Pastor," she commanded.

"Of course," I said, and decided upon a generic prayer for health and safety.

But no sooner had I grasped her hand, closed my eyes, and begun, "Let us pray," than she began growling in deep voice:

"*SATAN! SATAN! GET AWAY FROM ME, SATAN!*"

Everyone in the ED—patients and staff—spun around to see how I was torturing this poor psychotic woman.

My eyes snapped open as I let go of her hand, gently, and backed away from her. "It's OK. I'm your chaplain, your minister— here to help—but I'm going to let you rest now," I said, ready to run.

She asked me to pray again. Once more I stepped close only to meet her "*SATAN! SATAN! GET THEE BEHIND ME, SATAN!*"

Back to square one.

We went through this cycle three times before I told her I needed to check on another patient ("Mrs. Dirtbike"), whom I hoped had returned from her smoke break.

As I walked by the ED staff desk, the unit manager whispered: "I am *so* sorry." He felt terrible for asking me to check on her.

But I knew this was my job as a resident chaplain: to hold the space, no matter how terrifying, uncomfortable, or awkward. I was the buffer and connector between hospital staff and patients, patients and families—and, sometimes, life and death.

In those first weeks, I was taught to assess the crisis, listen intently, glean clues from the conversation to frame any theological context, notice opportunities for care, offer tools for coping, and reflect what I heard—authentically, with appropriate language.

At age 25, I learned how to be the competent death chaplain... and, apparently, Satan.

MICU

All hospital intensive care unit rooms—including MICU—have the same lighting. It's an iridescent purple gray, splashed with whatever the weather has to offer.

Two smells duel it out in these spaces: "anti-bacterial *everything*" and the stench of decay.

The soundtrack of an ICU such as MICU is a steady rhythm of beeps and clinical whispers, a "mixed and scratched" script of medical jargon. Patients are the lead actors in storylines for which they did not audition.

There's a hospital reality called "ICU psychosis." If an intensive care patient regains enough consciousness to be at all aware of their surroundings, they may become disoriented by the light, the smell, the beeps, the whispers, the odd time-keeping. Losing one's mind in the ICU is a reasonable reaction to being held health-hostage in a place where time is measured by data and the whisper, "Is the patient progressing?"

In any ICU—but especially MICU—when the body is beyond recovery and mechanical assistance is purposely withdrawn, the hospital's best and brightest are bedside to attempt control of any disturbing symptoms leading up to death. Chaplains call these helper-doctors "Geese," because of the way they swoop in with white coats, migrating from family to family to explain how and why bodies die. In environments such as the MICU, the seasoned doctors have the experience and skills to convey deep empathy and tenderness for the patients they long to save but know they can't. At the very least, they promise families they will do all they can to ensure a peaceful death.

As was the case with Lily.

My First Death

Lily Smith* had struggled her entire life with a disease that left her entire body—including her vital organs—compromised. Her condition made her physically weak, but spiritually brave. I was in my third week of the residency when I met Lily and her family. I didn't know it when I met her, but Lily would be the first person I ever saw die.

The Smiths were a rural family of "God talkers," cheery country folk who peppered every sentence with an invocation of "But the Lord." They reminded me of my own upbringing in a small town, where Christians exude a hopeful faith, outcomes are simple, and *everything*—including health outcomes—are dependent upon God. The Smiths felt like home.

For years, Lily had been confined to a wheelchair, now plastered with Jesus stickers. She was a small-town evangelist whose every minute had been dedicated to reminding others of how much God loved them. She'd been admitted to the MICU for an acute infection, one that required elephant-gun doses of medication and careful monitoring from ICU physicians. Lily was a rarity in MICU-land: one of our only "walkie-talkies"— exhausted, but conscious enough to converse.

Lily drew the MICU staff to her with a magnetic personality. Even those who had affinity for neither Jesus nor religion enjoyed caring for her and checking in.

"We'll be outta here in a few days, Chaplain," the Smiths would conclude. "You just keep prayin' for us."

"Of course," I would nod.

I visited Lily and the Smiths in the MICU every day over the course of several weeks. On a Wednesday afternoon, we'd had an especially upbeat conversation and connection. I felt buoyed with hope as I left the MICU and began making my way to catch the bus home. Then I heard the female hospital operator calmly sing, "Code Blue, Medicine Intensive Care Unit." She said it in an eerily professional way I assumed they must teach in hospital

* Not the patient's real name and details about the patient's condition and family come from what I experienced with several patients.

intercom school in order *not* to startle hospital visitors, patients, and families about the fact that *death is coming.*

Damn, I thought, turning back from the hospital exit and my route to the bus.

I returned to the MICU, where I anticipated that one of my more critical patients was already in their last hours. But the MICU doors opened to reveal a protective bulwark of Geese around *Lily's* bed—attending physicians, residents, and fellows screaming orders and interventions.

You Learn to Read the Signs

Cardiac and respiratory arrests ("codes") are nothing like medical TV drama portrayals. There are no dry, clean, chiseled people in pristine scrubs shouting well-formed dialogue. There are frantic, sweaty physicians and nurses, moving at warp speed and yelling staccato commands through surgical masks. Overflowing crash carts with heart defibrillators and resuscitation medications are destroyed by fistfuls of grabs. Ribs break, fluids fly, and each second counts.

When I realized it was Lily coding, I stood against the wall, shocked. I had no ability to pray. My only thought was: *Do her parents know?*

At some point, I heard the shout, "Where's the chaplain?" from the head fellow, as he peered above the chaos.

"I'm here," I yelled, my hand halfway raised like a timid middle schooler. He looked worried behind his wire-rimmed glasses. His frosty blue eyes seemed to say, *just in case,* then he put his head down and returned to his work.

The doctor didn't know my name, but he knew my title and credentials. "Clickety-Shoes," was the name my fellow chaplains have given *him,* for his ridiculous pretentious leather Italian shoes that screamed, "The Doctor is *IN!*"

But now Dr. Clickety-Shoes was a Brooks Brothers commercial in time-lapse, and I desperately wanted him to save Lily. I asked God to disregard my disdain for his shoes, which I now hoped would give him super powers.

Five minutes later, he breezed passed me. "Come with me," he directed. We walked down the corridor to the family consultation room, where the Smiths were huddled in terror.

"She's back," he said when he walked in, as if Lily had just gone for a Thai lunch—not as if this declaration would explode their world.

But I *still* admired him for what he *wasn't* saying, which was the sheer excellence with which he and his ICU team had just worked for nearly an hour—validating one of their miracle passes, issued directly from Jesus.

A steady stream of medical questions from the Smiths followed. He answered them with a precision that impressed all of us. He explained that, yes, Lily *had* been stable during her infection recovery, but she stopped breathing suddenly (respiratory code), most likely from the ongoing chronic disease that had already compromised her body. As he spoke he delivered his care notes in a well-versed package he'd rehearsed for all codes—only this time he added a line he didn't usually get to say: she was *still* alive.

He explained that the outlook was still very bleak—as she had been clinically *dead,* resuscitated, and now her breathing was being fully supported by a machine. His underlying message seemed to be: "We barely made it through this, and we don't yet know what the cognitive effects will be." Leaving, he turned toward me and nodded, as if to say: *Your turn.*

Patients and families who've experienced such dramatic, terrifying medical events have brushed against a spiritual cheese grater. Their substance is intact, but it's been shredded, and it will never fully recover its former form.

The door closed. I was left to hold whatever reasonable traumatic emotions and reactions the Smiths might or might not have—from joy of the miracle, to concern for the prognosis.

"Our Lily is alive," they rejoiced. "It's a miracle!"

As a newbie chaplain, CPE instruction for this situation was simple: be present, listen, and don't try to answer any large existential, medical, or theodicy questions. Repeat what you hear; comfort with whatever tool is appropriate.

"You think she'll be all right, Chaplain?"

"They're taking excellent care of her," I said.

"Will she make it?"

"I think we will know more soon," I said. Then I added, "I think we should pray for strength for her and us"—my amateur catch-all escape for the enthusiastically religious with questions for which none of us had answers.

"Will you go with us to visit her?" they asked.

They wanted back in the ring; they wanted to fight for Lily *with* her.

I followed protocol. "Let me check to see if they are ready for us."

MICU and other hospital staff implored chaplains to comfort and keep families occupied as long as possible after a code to give them time to clean up the mess, which looks nothing like the tidy set of *Grey's Anatomy*. No family should have to see the underbelly of what it takes to *literally* save a human life.

At the team's signal, we returned to the room to find Lily cleaned up, tucked in, and resting angelically in her bed with an endotracheal tube placed down her throat, connected to a ventilator. No longer bubbly, she was sedated and tranquil—looking like nothing you'd expect from someone who has just touched death and returned.

Her parents rubbed her hands and face, dropping in and out of prayers and Bible verses, pleading, "Please Jesus, help our baby."

I stayed a while, then left to give them time together. My chest was tight with secondary trauma from the Smiths' and my own shock.

One time, someone asked me what I did as a chaplain. "I hold things," I said. I was like a Tupperware container for their joy, sorrow, uncertainty, and the unknown.

Life-and-Death Decisions

When I arrived in the unit the next morning, Lily's room was busy with hushed movement. Her parents were still by her side, wearing the same clothes, eyes red with dark circles—indications that the nurses had allowed them to stay overnight. Strict overnight visitation rules were only lifted for patients not doing well.

"How is she?" I asked the nurse before I went in.

She pulled me out of their view, concerned. Per protocol, the night shift doctors and nurses had checked Lily's ventilator and sedation often.

Lily had responded *very well* to all her neuro-function tests, which surprised everyone.

While Lily's cognitive function was extraordinary, her respiratory response was not. When she had awakened, the doctors had turned down the ventilation settings, but her already compromised lungs had not responded well, indicating serious damage. When they had tried again, later, during another period of wakefulness, Lily had used grimaces, groans, and sign language to insist on the full removal of the breathing tube—her life source—even as her parents patiently explained to Lily *all* that had happened in the past 18 hours, and that the tube would likely have to stay in—perhaps even permanently through a tracheotomy.

Anxiety, groans, poor respiratory news, and Lily's requests for tube pulling (the denial of which led to a rather upset patient) had encapsulated this nurse's first one-and-a-half hours with Lily that morning. Lily, who had lived the life of a chronically sick person, was now immobilized for her own good, stuffed with plastic, breathing artificially, and recovering from a clinical death.

You learn to read the clues.

Thursday and Friday became a blur, because the signs were clear.

The infection Lily arrived with was now the least of everyone's concern. Her disease, compounded by the code, was claiming the basic functions she needed to survive—including breathing on her own. Medical professionals can cash in miracle cards with heroic resuscitation tactics, but they cannot defeat death's summons.

"Out," she mouthed clumsily during her neurological and respiratory checks.

"But if we take out the tube, baby, you won't be able to breathe," her mother pleaded each time. She stopped short of saying: *You will die, baby.*

During every shift for two days, the scene remained on repeat: Lily would try to tell everyone what she already knew: she didn't want to live confined to a wheelchair *and* a breathing tube. She would rather die.

Dr. Clickety-Shoes and his team assessed and reassessed. Was her brain *fully* functioning? Did she understand the connection between intubation and the ventilator keeping her alive? Did she *really* comprehend that without breathing assistance, she would die? Shift after shift, neurological tests and consultations with various medical staff yielded the same result: *yes, Lily understood.*

She knew from the beginning that her debilitating disease would one day consume her fragile frame and her vital organs. She knew that children born with her disease usually didn't even live to be a quarter-century old.

Two days after her code, Clickety-Shoes and the MICU team affirmed what Lily had been telling us all along: the tube and the artificial life-support must be removed—because, that's what the terminally ill, adult patient of sound mind wanted.

Word spread on the MICU quickly; everyone was simultaneously stunned—and impressed with her courage. The young woman from the hills of North Carolina who'd come in for an acute respiratory infection had gone from being a big fish in a little pond to a heartbreaking hero of a prestigious university medical center's intensive care unit. We began asking ourselves: *Would I make the same decision? Would I be this brave?* Later, I realized it was the way Mom felt when she repeated her "no knives" mantra. Day after day, even as surgeons begged her to consider surgery, as it was the way to delay her final day, she was clear: *"No knives."*

But the Smiths—like many other family members who find themselves in the midst of something similar—were not ready. They were praying for one last miracle. That miracle, Dr. Clickety-Shoes insisted, was not in the cards. Lily, though fully conscious and cognitively able, would never breathe without assistance again. My mother, though fully conscious and cognitively able, would not survive without surgery.

The Friday after Lily's code, my shift ended, and I said goodbye to the Smiths for the weekend, my heart crushed.

I'd only been home one hour, sulking in my pajamas with Mom and drowning myself in mindless sitcoms, when the MICU called.

"They want to extubate tonight," the nurse said. Her voice was confident; I realized that Lily had finally convinced her parents it was time. "They want you here," the nurse continued. "Can you come? We'll wait for you."

Of course I could come.

I returned to the hospital with one thought on my mind: *Why not ask the on-call chaplain? I was only a few weeks into this residency. Did they know I had never actually seen anyone die, let alone assisted with care at the end-of-life?*

Eleven years later—during the same Carolina August heat, I'd realize why: Lily and the Smiths chose *me* so that God could begin to prepare me to be with my mother.

The Perfect Death

"It's time," Dr. Clickety-Shoes said when he spotted me. It was late; he was staying past his shift to usher Lily to her new destination—a duty he could have easily transferred to his on-call colleagues, but chose not to. He was the one who had led his team to do all they could to bring her back to life, and now he wanted to ensure she had a peaceful death.

I walked in the room to hear Mrs. Smith plead with her daughter one last time, "Lily, are you sure, baby? You sure this is what you want?"

Lily nodded, her wiry fingers motioning to the thick plastic tube forcing her breaths. "Out," she mouthed again, firm.

The nurse and Dr. Clickety-Shoes ushered the herd of visitors into the hallway while they removed Lily's breathing tube. Then, they hailed us back in, and we moved to our positions. The Smiths insisted I stand at the foot of the bed, to conduct an informal "homegoing." Dr. Clickety-Shoes stood at the head of the bed, poised to monitor Lily closely for any symptoms and administer morphine to keep her pain- and distress-free.

The tubes were gone; she was surrounded by people caring for her. And Lily smiled the widest I seen her smile since she'd arrived.

My sweaty hands gripped my leather-bound travel Bible. I read what I knew the Smiths wanted to hear:

A reading from the prophet Isaiah, chapter 40, verse 31:
"But they that wait upon the LORD shall renew their strength;
they shall mount up with wings as eagles; they shall run,
and not be weary; and they shall walk, and not faint."
[Isa. 40:31–32, KJV]

"Let us pray," I said.

I don't know what I prayed then, but whatever the words the Holy Spirit placed in my mouth, what my heart cried was this:
God, I don't know what I'm doing. I've never seen anyone die. Help me to say the right thing for this family. I'm not certain how or why I'm here, or what I can do. Come, Holy Spirit. Be quick.

"Amen," I said, punctuating my actual and internal prayers.

I opened my eyes to see Clickety-Shoes jerking his head to attention, wavy hair bouncing—an indication that he'd been praying with us.

Mrs. Smith began to sing softly, and I looked at each face in the circle. This dying young woman had one last testimony to share; she'd brought us all together to witness that this earthly existence is not all there is, and that she was brave and courageous and confident that God awaited her, and would await us, too, one day.

We are born. We will die.

I don't remember if Lily was ever able to even take a breath on her own, but I do remember her smile. Mrs. Smith's singing grew softer as Lily's skin turned a dusky rose.

And then I saw it.

The hint of remaining color faded from her lips. In mere seconds, she turned pale, her hands cooled to the touch. Her essence—what had made Lily, Lily for over two decades, escaped from her worn-out shell. Whatever it was—her soul perhaps—hovered in the room with us for a sacred second—one in which, on the most primitive level—I *felt*, like a tiny butterfly wing fluttering against my heart.

And then she was gone.

We stood silently around the bed, bound by our common humanity and our common end.

It was the first time I'd seen anyone die.

And it was the perfect death.

I remember Lily's summer evening death. I remember its clarity, start to finish, and understood, as far as I was able, that I wanted to help provide a good death for others.

And though I couldn't know it at the time, it was the fertile ground from which I offered its fruitful lessons to my mother 11 years later.

Chapter 4

The King and Great One

*"Someone I loved once gave me a box full of darkness. It took
me years to understand that this, too, was a gift."*
—Mary Oliver

*"Our lives are not our own; from womb to tomb,
we are bound to others, past and present,
and by each crime and every kindness we birth our future."*
—David Mitchell, Cloud Atlas

Three years after my year-long hospital residency as the death
chaplain ended, I found myself sitting in a familiar Midwestern
church pew. Two hours west of Indianapolis, where corn grows
for miles, my father—an infamous tale-weaver, drug abuser, drug
dealer, and drug trafficker known in those parts as "The King"—
was laid out in a wooden coffin.

"King" was dressed in the only suit he ever "owned,"
borrowed from his father. My father's beard was long and curly,
neatly trimmed above his crossed arms that rested on his hand-
me-down pinstripes. King's youngest brother, "Boot," kneeled on
one knee in front of the coffin as if to genuflect to royalty. He
draped his arm over the edge and slipped unidentified objects
into the white lining of my father's final bed.

An hour later, Boot would burst through the Dana, Indiana,
Firehouse—the community of 600 people's only gathering

place—holding a portable karaoke machine. His attempt to further eulogize my father with terms such as "prophet" made the crowd collectively roll their eyes and crank up their reception conversations to a rowdy volume. Defeated, Boot finally sat back down to his fried chicken.

Such was life and death among my patriarchal lineage. A father whom I barely knew, laid in a casket we never expected to see him in. We had all imagined King as invincible and immortal, eternally young, fueled by a life of illegal uppers and downers, shirking any responsibility that sought to tie him down.

Because he had already lived so long and so hard, his death seemed impossible. He'd defied the odds time after time, from his hearse-driving, draft-dodging days to cross-country shenanigans, from extreme poverty to inheritance; surviving motorcycle accidents and chronic diseases while talking his way out of any law-breaking endeavor. The safest bet we'd all felt we could ever make was that he'd outlive us all, which was why *none* of us imagined we'd line the pews of Dana Community Bible Church to eulogize the man Vermillion County had thought to be invincible.

It was one of many reasons I'd written him a scathing letter the December before his June death on the injustice of *my* trauma caused by *him*, rescinding an invitation for my upcoming July wedding. He dropped dead a month before my mother walked me down the aisle.

My father was a complex character. A small-town celebrity who fancied himself an Orthodox Jew with a Protestant affinity for Jesus and a Catholic reverence for Mary, he suffered from schizo-affective disorder, while also manifesting other related mental illnesses—such as mania and depression—as well. Though raised in the Dana Community Bible Church, he still swore our family was Jewish, and that some shameful person had switched our name from "Jewman" to "Lewman" to protect us from the anti-Semites of rural Indiana. One learned quickly to take King's stories with a grain of salt.

As far as I know, my blue-eyed, fair-skinned paternal *grandfather* was of German descent. But my *father* did *look* different from the family tribe, as do I. He had olive skin and dark hair that curled when he grew it long. His hazel eyes had striking gold edges. He certainly could have passed for Jewish, and tried his best to do so.

But the metal crucifix he super-glued to the dashboard of every vehicle he ever owned gave him away, as did the three-foot statue of Mary Magdalene in his front yard.

The King was born, raised, and died in rural Indiana. He was a son of a farmer and a small-town entrepreneur. When my parents divorced when I was six, my father slipped back into the Midwestern identity he felt most comfortable in: overalls, holey t-shirts, an unruly long beard, shoulder-length black hair, and a Yankees ball cap.

Since adolescence, King had been known for swinging swiftly from one end of the spectrum to the other: from a brilliant professional—he held a master's degree in recreational therapy—to a disheveled vagabond who sounded like one of his psychiatric patients. The people of Dana and nearby townships revered his antics and soaked up his embellished stories. Because he was dubbed "The King" at an early age, and signed every return address envelope to me with it (King), we had it engraved on his tombstone.

The King never met a stranger; his entourage was thick with men whose street names mimicked animal parts and cities, some of whom spent years in federal prison—or, as my father put it, "joined the circus."

My strained relationship with The King had been brewing since my parents divorced. The letter was a culmination of decades of stuffed, internalized anger and pain. Supporters of my assertiveness in asking him not to attend our wedding celebrated my bravery. Those fiercely loyal to him gave me hell. The letter was impulsive, but felt appropriate at the time. I had been seeing a therapist who was administering EMDR (Eye Movement Desensitization Reprocessing), a therapeutic intervention for those who've experienced trauma. I was eager to avoid confrontation and embarrassment at my upcoming nuptials.

It was my mother who'd raised me fulltime since age six, and I wanted to celebrate her and the countless cheerleaders—including family, friends, teachers, and mentors—who'd nurtured me into adulthood. My father had certainly had *a hand* in my maturation, but in a trauma-has-made-me-resilient sort of way. I was prejudiced against his schizo-affective disorder that he couldn't cure, and didn't want his paranoia and antics to embarrass me and distract from those who'd been my stable rocks all along. So, I revoked my father's wedding invitation on December 2, 2009. We never spoke again. Six months later, he died.

If my crystal ball hadn't been broken that week, I would have placed that letter in a drawer and let it be. But I was *certain* King would outlive all of us, as he'd laughed in the devil's face so many times already, and the consequences of fast-living never seemed to catch up with him.

The letter felt like my best option for a temporary reprieve to get through my wedding sanely and celebrate those family and friends who deserved the real credit for getting me there.

I never had the chance to apologize, reconcile, or say goodbye to him. The finality of it is smothering.

King's death was so unlike my MICU patients' deaths, and my mother's. Though my brain would have me believe that I can *control* and *plan* a good death for myself and others—peacefully dying in a hospital or hospice, or at home, surrounded by light and love beaming from adoring faces, the reality is: death is not always tidily bookended and convenient. We can die anywhere, anytime—and alone.

I had not anticipated my father's end would arrive this way: a cardiac arrest on a June day, followed by a fall in which he hit his head and lay there till he was discovered by a friend who'd come over to mow his lawn. Because I've experienced many deaths, including those of my own parents, people often ask me which is harder: a long (or short) personal goodbye with a terminally ill loved one, or a swift death in which there is no time to say anything.

Time after time, the latter has struck me as the most unfair.

As with my MICU patients and families, my heart was shredded by the spiritual cheese grater, and would not return to its former wholeness. With my mother's death, there had been time (though brief) to tie up loose ends. She was too weak to have an existential chat, but she knew I was there. My father had had no one in those last moments of consciousness before a rural ambulance carted him off to Clinton Hospital to put him on a ventilator in time for my aunt and uncle to arrive. Life support was withdrawn, and there was no goodbye from me. I received a call afterward, when all was said and done.

My father's death left me feeling like a sealed envelope. Our memories, talks, and chapters were folded and tucked inside, a dotted timeline whose finality was sealed with a wax stamp, never to be opened on this side of heaven.

Sudden Death

A year after my father was lowered into the ground at Bono cemetery, just outside Dana, Indiana, Fred's father suffered a cardiac arrest during my in-laws' family reunion.

It was a Friday night in June, the one-year anniversary of my father's death. Fred's father had invited his parents, brothers, sister, and all the kids to his lake house for the weekend.

That afternoon, "Great One" (that's what I called him) had taught me how to crack and eat crab legs. He found it humorous that I found it disgusting, and he teased me for my queasiness. After a crab leg or two, I went upstairs to wash the smell off my hands. I never saw him conscious again. None of us did.

Thirty minutes later, having recovered from my queasiness enough to leap into chaplain mode, I offered to take a turn giving CPR. Watching the scene unfold, I began to discern clues, read the signs. And somehow, I knew how his story would end—like Lily's: code blue, life support, withdrawal, goodbye.

Three days later, Fred, his mother, his brother, and I were by Great One's bedside, removing life support from a 53-year-old man who'd been struck by a "widow-maker" heart attack, the blockage of a main artery whose symptoms are often overlooked or silent.

I have played the role of death chaplain many times, but that day I was right back where I started with Lily, nervously ensuring that Great One had a meaningful, sacred transition from here to eternity.

The Great One

The second death of a parent in one year sent a wave of shock through our marriage. I was still recovering from my own father's death—and Fred's father's passing reignited and compounded my grief. Our contrasting personal and theological perspectives on death and afterlife (Christian for me; Hindu for Fred) made navigating grief tricky. We shuffled clumsily through the dark path of sudden loss.

Our fathers led very different lives. Both were well-educated, stoic and stubborn, and, at times, distant and unreadable. They shared a common ending, but the journey that led each of them there was distinct.

Fred Edward Eaker Sr. was far from the showboat of tall-tale-telling schizo-affective disorder the King had been. Fred's father was quiet, steadfast, and responsible; a proud mechanical engineer and provider who enjoyed tinkering with machines, fishing, and piddling on the home slot machine he had purchased on eBay.

I called him "Great One" because everyone in my paternal family shows affection by bestowing nicknames.

"What should I call you?" I asked him, shortly after we met.

"O Great One," he replied, in the deadpan humor he was known for.

"That settles it," I responded.

Great One was an accomplished mechanical engineer in the dry foods industry. He worked hard and did well by his family. Fred's father could fix *anything*. He brought old boats back to life and onto the water, and put socks in carburetors to return vehicles to the highway. Great One was also famous for drinking a gallon of milk every 48 hours, and loved Las Vegas—where he always won big.

"How do you do it?" I asked, wanting to know his gambling secret.

"I *listen* to the machines," he said, in all seriousness.

When my father died, I envied Fred's access to his father and the steadfastness Great One offered his family. I didn't know such fathers existed. And I sometimes neglected to empathize with the fact that sometimes having a *present* parent can be just as complicated as having an absent one. Fred's relationship with his father was often tense. Great One rarely showed emotion, and lacked patience in teaching his boys. The contemplative thoughtfulness that made Fred a stellar priest and monk met Great One's machine-mindedness with strain. Fred's father's communication style could be stern; his take-charge attitude left a young Fred feeling inferior and inadequate. They argued over Fred's adolescent exploration of Eastern philosophy. Ultimately, Fred's conversion to Hinduism built a wall between them.

But things had thawed out when Fred and I began dating. Great One and the entire family inhaled Easter hope when they found out Fred was dating a Baptist minister. They imagined little

Freddy might return to the Christian fold—or, at the very least, find more balance as a religious minority living in the Bible Belt with a "good, Protestant woman" by his side. Their father-son tension also loosened with Fred's blossoming success in his IT career. As talented as Great One was, he relied on Fred for tech support, which made Fred feel valued and accomplished.

Ensuring a Good Birth

When Fred's father died, we were all together. Unlike with my father's death, we were with Great One every step of the way—from his cardiac arrest to his withdrawal from life support.

Because I wasn't in Indiana for my own father's cardiac arrest, it was surreal to be so close to Great One's. Four years after my residency, my father-in-law's mysterious code ignited all the skills I learned at the hospital—and, in an instant, I was back in the ICU, in a chaplain-as-translator role. Only, this time I was in this strange space of playing dual roles: the chaplain *and* the wife of the bereaved.

It was one of *my people* on life support; it was *my person* whose prognosis was grim. But I knew the moment I saw Great One unconscious on his bed with purple, oxygen-deprived skin where we'd be three days later. I'd lived it for an entire year. *Cardiac arrest. Ambulance resuscitation. Emergency Department stabilization. Ventilators. Pressors. Intensive Care Unit. Decisions…*

Courageous doctors tell you it's a "wait-and-see" game. I know what is left unsaid in those words: "Your loved one is *never* coming back." Nonetheless, options are detailed, decisions discussed, life support withdrawn…and, then, death arrives. *Repeat.* I knew the cycle so well I could anticipate every move the medical personnel made, and every reaction Fred's family would have.

I returned to the role without missing a beat. I spoke with doctors and nurses, explained my training, and requested their transparency in Great One's prognosis. They seemed relieved; I translated medicalese for them in family room meetings, just as I had in the MICU with Dr. Clickety-Shoes. They relied on me to bridge the gap, to be the liaison from the medical to the emotional. In that role of chaplain and helper, I didn't have to confront my own grief bubbling up every hour as Fred's father inched closer to death.

I encouraged Fred to express all I hadn't been able to share with my father: love, apologies, forgiveness, assurance, gratitude, and goodbyes.

Months later, devastated by Great One's death, I merged it with my own father's death, such that I was grieving two men I barely knew, but two men I had so desperately wanted to love me. I'd had Great One as a father-in-law for only one year, and I had taken it for granted that he'd be with us for decades.

When Great One died, I realized just how much Fred and I grappled with their deaths—and our subsequent grief—in different ways. In my Christian head and heart, I played by the theology of YOLO (You Only Live Once). My father had lived his *one* life—and it was now gone. But in Fred's Hindu view, our fathers were now living *new* lives—and had already lived—millions of lives.

It was a lesson in theology and in pastoral care: each loss—and the subsequent interpretation of afterlife—is unique. Inasmuch as our religious and spiritual traditions assign doctrinal assertions to our ultimate purpose ("Where are we going?"), grief impacts us on the individual level. Our loved one is no longer physically present with us, and we grapple with this—and make meaning out of it—in different ways.

YOLO is what made my father's unexpected death so difficult to process. He'd had one shot to be my father; I'd had one shot to be his daughter. We both screwed up royally, and so his absence was paralyzing.

If I consider Fred's Hindu YALO (You Actually Live On) theology of reincarnation, my father's soul is out *there* or *here* somewhere, reincarnated as perhaps a grumpy goat or budding truck driver, and here I am, left behind—and stuck in his past.

Following my father's death, Fred comforted me in all the ways a loving spouse does. He traveled with me to rural Indiana for the funeral, helped me clean out my father's trailer, and anticipated anything I needed. I *needed* Fred's strength; he was my heart and brain to help make decisions when I had no bandwidth. Most of all, he was now my very own chaplain presence: holding my anger, sadness, and denial.

This steady, emotional comfort helped me survive the 30 days between King's death and our wedding. That month was the one break in our typically nonstop theological chattering, the bond that drew us even closer together, like magnets. I didn't want to think about the effect navigating two faith traditions would have on my future grief—I just wanted to survive my wedding.

After we were married, and the buzz of celebration subsided, grief returned to the forefront. I began to wonder if my father had made it to heaven. I imagined God with unlimited mercy, even claiming someone as frustrating and exhausting as The King. Yet the bereaved don't necessarily want their loved ones in heaven. We want them here—a part of the familiar landscape in which we've always known them. No one wants to be surprisingly and tragically separated too soon from their children, partners, parents, or best friends—especially not in sudden ways that leave many things unsaid. Grief is for the living, and living loved ones want their people back.

I wanted my father back.

Months after Dad died, I questioned everything. I cracked the door to theological conversation with Fred about my father's afterlife: was it the traditional Christian linear path I imagined it to be, or could it possibly be Hinduism's cyclical journey, from one life to the next?

Because Fred grew up in a nominally Christian family, he was versed in Christianity's linear, progressive journey: he knew about the fall of Adam and Eve (humanity's original sin), salvation through Jesus, baptism, and one-way tickets to heaven. He also knew that the denominational nuances along the Christian path are wide and varied, but the essence remains the same: it is a linear journey from point A to point B.

But Fred's later study of Hinduism, his monasticism, and, ultimately, his ordination as a Hindu priest meant he no longer believed in the linear journey. "We have been born and died innumerable times," he'd tell me, quoting Hindu scripture.

I'd respond, "But why would we want to do this all over again, learning [or re-learning] the same lessons?

Our conversations on our differing theologies of the afterlife made it clear to me that while our partners, family, and friends can be of great comfort in our grief, they can also hold very different understandings of what happens after life. Therefore, they assign different meanings to what it means to live without the departed. We cannot expect those closest to us to experience the loss in the same way we do.

Doubt

Four years after Dad's death, Fred and I attended a winter conference on the spiritual practices of the early Christian church. Fred was there for the theological and academic heft; I was there to glean any emotional wisdom I could from the desert mothers and fathers.

At the beginning of the day, participants were invited to pick up index cards with words written on them in big, bold permanent marker. My eyes shifted to the card that read: "DOUBT." It had been years since I'd been with the dying, but the cadence of grief remained, and its questions lingered. "DOUBT": Life, death, grief, afterlife—what did it all *really* mean?

I don't remember much of the workshop content, just those black letters, inked permanently on my card. During breaks, I stuffed myself with peanut M&Ms and cheap cinnamon rolls while Fred was eager to parse what he had learned about the early church and his critique of the way Christianity does things *now*. It was the first intense theological setting Fred and I had been in together in which we were both students. I realized then just how different our views of faith were. Doubt came riding in, gaining its welcome from a damn index card.

Since Fred had studied Hinduism's framework, and also had a deep respect for early church writers and thinkers, he would forever question the gilded theology of heaven Christianity landed on, and I was still wrapping my head around reincarnation. Fred and I had traveled to Hindu monasteries and spent countless hours studying scripture; I'd even written a book about our interfaith marriage. But we hadn't yet taken the time to examine, in depth, our different perspectives on life after death until blindsided by the loss of these two men.

When we arrived home from the retreat, I ran for the shower—which is where I go when I want to be alone, warm, and safe. Back during my death chaplain year, I always showered as soon as I walked through the door, home from the hospital. I couldn't breathe again until I rinsed the chaos and smell of death down the drain. But MICU chaplaincy days had closure: they could be washed away. Our fathers' deaths; lingering waves of grief; and these interfaith questions of heaven, reincarnation, and the afterlife—these were not so easily forgotten.

My mother always said that when her babies—me and Ron—cried hard, we gasped uncontrollably for air between fits. It came up through our throats with a gurgling; our lips pouted out and trembled, in what my mother named the "snubs." Snubs cannot be replicated under normal conditions. It's ugly, hard crying—such that your face contorts and you realize this is going to be rough, but you're going to have to push through, because you'll feel better once you've cried as hard as you can for as long as you can.

I snubbed through my shower after that workshop. My sadness was so uncontrollable that I was wretched.

"Why, God? Why are you doing this to me?" *Why would you take both our fathers away from us at such a young age?* I mouthed a silent scream, remembering the "DOUBT" card, and how much doubt I felt about my grief, my father's destination, and which path—Christianity's linear or Hinduism's cyclical—was "right."

I glided my hands through my wet hair and opened my eyes.

Fred was standing there, shower curtain pulled away, watching me. *Smiling.* He'd seen my silent monologue, my Job-like lament, cursing the day I was born and wallowing in my doubt.

"Go away!" I screamed and threw my wash cloth at him.

I needed room to grieve.

I needed room to doubt.

Even Jesus gave Thomas room. I wanted time and space to question the *whys* of our fathers' deaths. Why had our fathers so abruptly been taken away, and where had they gone?

Chapter 5

Say Hello to Heaven

"This life is tottering like a drop of water on a lotus petal."
—*Govinda dāsa Kavirāja, Bhajahŭ Re Mana,*
Sri Gaudiya-Gita Guccha

I don't know what God is.
I don't know what death is.
But I believe they have between them
some fervent and necessary arrangement.
—*Mary Oliver, "Sometimes," Red Bird*

There's more than one answer to these questions
Pointing me in a crooked line
And the less I seek my source for some definitive
The closer I am to fine.
—*Amy Elizabeth Ray and Emily Ann Sallers,*
"Closer to Fine"

Ultimate Purpose

In the World Religions college courses I teach, I encourage my students to approach each tradition using three questions that anchor academic study of religion: What is the "Ultimate Reality"? What is the "Way of Life"? What is the "Ultimate Purpose"?

Talking about the "Ultimate Purpose" always trips them up, for two reasons. First, they don't want to die, even though I remind them that the mortality rate is still 100 percent. Second, religious, spiritual, and indigenous traditions can often be unclear about *where*, precisely, we are going—and *why* we are here to begin with. At its core, the Ultimate Purpose is to assign meaning to the "Why are we here?" and "Where are we going?" questions.

Nearly every religious, spiritual, moral, ethical, and intellectual tradition has answers, definitions, and nuances for its Ultimate Purpose. Many traditions have formulated official doctrines that deeply consider death and the afterlife. On an individual level, chaplaincy taught me that practitioners of various faiths may fervently cling to, reject, bend, or adjust their tradition's doctrine and dogma when they are faced with death. Everyone interprets the "company line" in different ways—particularly at the end of life.

Rev. Sally Bates, retired Duke Divinity School chaplain and my supervisor following my hospital residency, told me that the key as the chaplain, or the friend, or the loved one, or the patient...is to be flexible, especially when the circumstance of the dying is unexpected and surreal.

In speaking about the times she's offered pastoral care at the end of life, Chaplain Bates named the conundrum ministers face when helping patients and families cope with the Ultimate Reality.

"What script are we using?" she said, "Which tab? Religious? Spiritual but not religious? Hope? Absurdity? Magical thinking? What is the meta-narrative, and what vocabulary list is most helpful?" Continuing, she also cautioned me to remember, "And so many times, the script flips."

"Open, open, open" had been the mantra I clung to as a hospital chaplain. I was not my patients' pastor; I hadn't had years to develop long-standing relationships with them, to know their frameworks concerning the afterlife—or what their faith of origin or choice had taught them. I learned to watch for breadcrumbs patients or families offered me, to listen for openings and opportunities to provide care. I had to be willing, as Sally advised, to use the vocabulary list that was most helpful for them, given what they did—or didn't—believe.

YOLO?

On the fourth Sunday of Advent a few years before my mother's death, Mom and I stood in the sunlit narthex of our church with Nora, a staunch octogenarian Baptist whose ruby red lipstick matched her beaded Christmas sweater.

The previous Sunday, she'd hollered out at us through the passenger window of her husband's sedan; she was delighted to see us heading to worship after mom's long home confinement due to declining physical health and chronic depression.

"My husband 'bout had a fit that I was hollerin' at y'all last week," she laughed. "He said, 'Quit hangin' out that window like a teenager!' I told him, 'I'm 82. I think I can do whatever I want,'" she said, before adding, "After all, we only go around once—" and then she paused, and looked at me with all seriousness, finishing with: "...or do we?" Then, she laughed.

"Who knows?" I offered.

"That's right," she confirmed. "We *don't* know, and that's the big question."

And there, on the Advent Sunday of Love, with five decades separating Nora and me, I realized that, because we *don't* know, it really does affect how we live. It might be the difference between hanging our 82-year-old limbs out the car window, skydiving, getting that enormous chest tattoo we've always wanted, eating as sumptuously as possible—or practicing mental discipline and limiting our desires, because equanimity is what counts if we want to land a better life next go-round. If we believe we've only got one chance, we may live on the edge. If we believe we've already done it before and we'll do it again, we may feel that nothing need be extreme or flamboyant.

One-Way Ticket, or Metro Card?

None of us can—or should—pretend to know the absolute *definitive* answer about the afterlife. But how do the world's religious traditions teach us to cope with the unknown? For Fred and me, our fathers' deaths one year apart flung us face-first into the question of Ultimate Purpose, to wonder if the destination was linear (a one-way ticket from here to heaven) or cyclical (with an infinite "metro card" for the cycle of reincarnation). We had two very different ideas and approaches that shaped our grief journeys and nearly tore us apart.

For me, the finality of my father's death cramped my heart and seized my breath when I realized I'd never ever see him on earth again. Christians rely on the linear path to heaven: we are born; somewhere along the line, we're saved, and thus (fingers crossed!) we get our one-way ticket. Heaven, though, didn't cut it for me. I wanted to see and talk with my Dad *here,* on earth, not some time later in some far-flung realm of celestial bodies. Plus, what if he didn't make it to heaven? What if I don't make it to heaven? And even if we should both land there, would we even still know each other, or have the same relationship we'd had *here* on earth, in life? I had far more questions than answers.

Fred, on the other hand, was confident and comforted by Hinduism's doctrine and theology of the afterlife: his father's soul merely shed its bodily shell, like changing into dry clothes after a swim. The essence of his father, his *soul,* still existed somewhere—maybe even among us, being born into a life determined by his karma. And *before* he was Fred's father, his soul had existed in many other physical forms—animal or human—over and over.

These diametrically opposed reactions to our fathers' deaths fostered loads of tears and frank conversations on Christian and Hindu approaches to what comes next. We grieved our losses in very different ways. When my Uncle Jon and Aunt Phyllis phoned me to tell me my father had died, I wailed. I clung to his metaphorical, and literal, coffin. It was sudden, visceral grief—physically nauseating, but brief. When Fred's father was withdrawn from life support four days after the family reunion cardiac arrest, Fred—with tear-filled eyes—quietly turned to God, chanting a soft Hindu mantra into his father's ear. Fred knew that *his* father was only *his* father temporarily and prayed that his father would now begin a new life, and that his father's journey toward fully belonging to God would continue.

I, on the other hand, was *pissed.* In all my "DOUBT," I'd shaken my fist at God in the shower, the word in *all caps,* in thick black ink from the index card of my heart. I had no definitive answers. I grieved loudly, quickly, and dramatically. Then, I internalized it, stuffing it all down until it came up the day I picked up that damn index card and I wondered where my father had gone, why he'd been plucked from me so young, and whether all this heaven stuff was for real.

Is Heaven for Real?

When I was a young teen, and before I even knew Christianity's official doctrinal stance on death and the afterlife, I wanted heaven to be just like *earth*, only without the yuck of landfills, wrinkles, flu, death, and taxes.

In my middle-school mind, my biggest concerns about heaven were: the guest list and the party agenda. I wanted heaven to be an exclusive club. I imagined that only people I liked would be there. None of my irritating schoolmates or history's villains would be admitted. I expected a cruise ship director God to provide a detailed list of daily activities and options—such as trampoline jumping and episodes of *The Young and the Restless*, as well as the dessert buffet times and choir rehearsals.

If you've ever endured a boring worship service, you understand the nagging heavenly priorities I had at age 13. How might it feel to spend *eternity* without life as we knew it to be on earth? When I thought about this question too much or too long, I'd have an existential crisis, so I pretended that heaven would be *only* the best parts of earth.

But this was just a sixth grader's Hallmark movie of afterlife: imagined pretty much as a rich girl's summer camp. It's not what Christian scripture, theology, and doctrine detail. Even when I was in seminary at Duke, I didn't *really* want to learn the intricacies of Christianity's views on heaven. I longed for the simple mystery of faith, the kind that filled country churches hidden among corn and tobacco fields. It was faith that one belted forth from the dark blue Baptist hymnals with broken spines, worn from rugged parishioners' hands longing for an hour of solace amid a hard life.

This was the sort of faith I'd learned about in my mother's and father's home church: You work, you get saved, you die, you hope—in the best-case scenario—to enjoy heavenly bliss.

But this is *not* the Christian Church's official stance. Though we certainly long for heaven to mirror earth, the Church says it probably doesn't. Even with a seminary degree, it's difficult for me to parse *precisely* what happens to Christians following death. This is mostly because all branches of Christianity *do not agree* on the specifics; nor is there one source, text, map, prophet, or doctrine that clearly outlines the step-by-step process, as in a YouTube tutorial.

Christian denominations remain heterogeneous on the major questions: Is there a *physical* heaven or hell? Is heaven metaphorical or symbolic for eternal union with (in the case of heaven)—or separation from (in the case of hell)—God? What about the Catholic doctrine of purgatory? How and where does bodily resurrection fit in? Judgement Day? Rapture? The Apocalypse? Soul Sleep?

What does the Bible *say* about our afterlives? It depends upon whom you ask. As with Facebook relationship status, it's complicated. I tell my students: if you locked three cradle Christians—a Greek Orthodox, a Roman Catholic, and a Southern Baptist—in a room until they unanimously agreed on the *specifics* of baptism and communion alone (much less something no living person has ever experienced—i.e., "the afterlife"), you're going to wait awhile. In fact, they may never come out.

This is to say that Christianity, much like the other global world religions—Judaism, Islam, Hinduism, and Buddhism— is a *very* large category. Under this umbrella lie varying views, doctrines, interpretations of scripture, opinions, and cultures surrounding what's in (orthodox) and what's out (heresy).

Heavenly Lessons

Perhaps the most compelling lessons on Ultimate Purpose I gleaned from my patients and my mother is this: when the time comes, don't worry about it so much. In the hospital deaths I've seen, I rarely saw patients or families frantic about *where* someone "was going." Rather, I experienced a mysterious assurance and hope. Patients didn't seem to fret about hell, nor dark destinations. If or when they did, they could easily be comforted with love, touch, prayers, and presence. Loved ones didn't seem to fret about judgment or doom for their people. They just wanted to love them while they were still here. Near the time of death, no one was too concerned with complex theological doctrine or what the Bible *really* says about heaven, hell, or the afterlife.

Instead, people leaned on "blessed assurance." They reached for the spiritual tools they'd learned as children—some of which they'd carried into adulthood. They prayed or asked for prayer— even if they weren't the praying type. They read light, encouraging verses of scripture, and told one another that Lily or Johnny or whoever was going to a better place, even if they weren't certain just what that place was. Patients, too, seemed at peace. When they were conscious, they spoke in metaphors and relished the peace and light that surrounded them. Their faces and bodies were relaxed, rarely on alert for the Grim Reaper.

To be sure, family members didn't want them to leave, and patients didn't necessarily want to go. But when it was clear that the end was imminent, there was an urgency to preserve those final days, hours, and moments for faithful encouragement and vocabulary that fit *their* life's script.

Chaplaincy taught me that when someone is actively dying, hardly anyone is ruminating on official church doctrine of the afterlife. At the bedside of a dying person who is imagining heaven to be just like the earthly good times they had with their now-deceased relatives, no empathetic seminary professor or chaplain worth their salt is going to say, "Well...actually, *that's heresy.*" Dying people want and need peaceful *reassurance* that a comforting afterlife awaits. They—and their families—want to know that they will not suffer unimaginable pain as they die. The dying also want the peace of knowing that the ones they physically leave behind will be OK. Most of all, they want to know and feel that people love them, that they will be remembered. They also want to know that God loves them and is ready to embrace them.

When doubt lingers, I lean on what my patients and mother taught me: death's approach is not the time to get preachy. When it comes to a linear shot to heaven or cycles of reincarnation, Nora summed it up best: we don't know, *really*.

But in my spiritually immature moments, I consider being an angel and worshiping God 24/7, *forever,* to be just a wee bit boring compared to all the social media stimuli I've enjoyed here on earth. Plus, I cannot picture my grumpiest dead relatives enjoying singing in the heavenly choir, when they hated it on earth. Most of all, I do not see my long-haired, long-bearded, overall-wearing, law-breaking King in a choir robe. I do, however, *see* him *hustling* the other angels, weaving tall tales, cutting in line at the buffet, and trying to talk God into letting him sit around smoking a *lot* of pot.

Is That You, Daddy?

North Carolina's annual state fair is 11 days of golden-fried deliciousness in the heart of October. This celebration of coronary disease beckons residents from our state's nooks and crannies to Raleigh, where agriculture becomes an excuse to consume a day's worth of calories in one funnel cake.

Four months after my father's June death, Fred and I stood in line at the Old Grist Mill, a small wooden structure nestled in the fairgrounds' "Village of Yesteryear." The rickety wood structure ground corn into cornmeal for sale, and lured would-be customers in with free hush puppies (the caviar of the South). Fred is a hush puppy fanatic, so we joined the long line that formed outside the shack and down the paved path.

Five people behind us in line, a man began to holler, "What are they a-doin' in there, grindin' the corn? This is a-takin' too long." I turned around.

The town crier was a tall, slender man with a long, white, scraggly beard and equally unkempt hair. His lose, faded overalls couldn't hide his ascites pot belly; he scratched his groin and pulled a red handkerchief from his back pocket and blew his nose.

It was my father, just as he would have looked and acted had he lived to be old enough to quit dying his beard *Just for Men* jet black.

"Hurry...it...up!" The man yelled through cupped hands. I elbowed Fred. "It's *him!*" I whispered. "Who?" He turned around to assess which *him* I could possibly be referring to. "Daddy!" I said.

Fred never met my father, but they talked on the phone once. Dad manically chatted nonstop for 20 minutes, telling Fred (the former monk) in his signature tall-tale way (lies) about how he (the King) was actually a monastic. When Fred, exhausted, handed the phone back to me, my father said, "That Fred is a talker! I couldn't get in a word—ha!"

Fred assessed the old man standing in line behind us. "It doesn't work that way," he laughed. "How does it work, then?" I asked, disappointed that my father's state fair reincarnation was being hijacked by theological details.

"First, he might not have come back as a human."

"What?"

"Depends on his karma."

"What would he be, then?"

"I dunno—an animal maybe."

"Do you think I'd recognize him if I saw him?"

"Probably not. You don't recognize anyone from your past life, do you?"

"You think I had a past life?"

"Of course. You've had a million of them."

This made my brain hurt.

"The soul is eternal. We only change bodies," Fred added, matter of factly, as if he were ordering kettle corn.

"I ain't gettin' no younger!" The old man yelled.

"Little does he know," Fred whispered.

I no longer felt compelled to wait for two free hush puppies. I pulled Fred out of line. "Daddy" was simultaneously exasperated and elated that two people had dropped out of line; his voice faded into the buzz of carnival rides as we walked away.

We settled on a chocolate-covered frozen banana and browsed the animals. I'd forgotten about reincarnation until I saw an old goat standing in a corner stall, separated from the others.

"Baaaaaaa," it shrieked at me, grumpy.

"Daddy, is that you?"

I realized I was experiencing what all the bereaved encounter: we are desperate for "our people" to live on, regardless of whether we've lost them abruptly. Specifically, since we've never existed in the world without our biological or adoptive parents until they have left us, the void we feel when they are gone is as real as that of a lost child at the state fair, searching for their mom and dad in a sea of people and livestock.

Is That You, Clark?

Even before Mom and Dad died, I'd had nagging feelings about life after death, and what a cold, terrible system it was to grow to love people so deeply, only to be separated from them.

Call me a heretic, but I don't think God thought this all the way through. Heaven or hell, purgatory or reincarnation, why wasn't there a better system for *keeping in touch* after death?

Maybe there is, and we just don't realize it—or perhaps we are so eager to make sense and meaning out of our finite mortal lives that we've invented ways to soothe ourselves: like that *nagging* way in which you *insist* you must have known someone "in another life" because you *immediately* have a bond with them that is otherwise illogical and unexplainable; or the way we call children with deep eyes and precocious vocabularies "old souls."

It's all mystical and mysterious, and we're stuck with human brains that cannot even begin to understand it all.

Nearly a decade ago, I was writing at a coffee shop—a hut, really—among the tall North Carolina pines, where I'd previously shared a meaningful conversation and caffeine with a seminary classmate named Clark. He was one of those people with whom you felt an *instant* connection, as if you had known him for years. A year previous to that day on which I was back there, writing, Clark had died unexpectedly in his sleep—at only age 29.

Now I sat alone at the table where we'd laughed years before—him, with his tall, lanky frame and his self-deprecating humor, and me with my awkward crush. I thought about him as I ladled heaps of sugar and regret in my coffee. I had never told Clark that he was the first friend I made in seminary, or that his encouragement was one of the many reasons why I hadn't dropped out when Duke's academic load nearly crushed me. I stirred my drink and I longed to see him one more time to tell him all *those* things—the things we wish we'd said to those who've left.

In that moment, a golden retriever arrived at my table, *inside* the coffee shop, sat dutifully next to me, and stared at me. It had no owner running after it. No other human in sight. No collar, nor leash. *Inside the shop.* I looked around to see if someone had poured me Iowaska instead of dark roast. But no one seemed alarmed or even noticed the dog. Not one person loved on him, as per usual when an irresistible canine is present.

I leaned over and whispered to the dog: "Is that you, Clark?"

My brain hadn't skipped a beat, as if it were not even my *own brain computing the possibility,* but *my soul seeing* my former classmate in a furry coat.

The dog blinked at me and wagged its talk.

"Oh my God, it *is* you, isn't it?" I said.

He wagged his tail again.

We stared at each other for a minute, and I silently told Doggy-Clark all the things I'd wanted to tell him when he was living. As soon as I finished the last sentence of my monologue, the dog got up and disappeared, just as randomly and swiftly as he'd sat tableside. My brain switched back to rational mode: *No... No way... It* couldn't *have been.*

As silly as it was, and as offended as some might be that I thought my friend had reincarnated into a dog (though *Clark* wouldn't have been *that* offended), that listening dog brought some healing, wherever he came from. For whatever reasons he popped up, I made meaning out of his presence, and that, too, is a way humans can process death, dying, and grief.

Real Talk: Theology in Everyday Life

The truth is that we can earn fancy theology degrees from Duke, Yale, Princeton, Harvard, or wherever, drowning ourselves in library books and orthodox theology on the proper doctrine of the afterlife, and it doesn't actually mean much—or help—when it comes time to do the hard work of watching someone die, experiencing a significant loss, and grieving loved ones. Brilliance falls flat in the face of death.

A seminary education isn't necessary—or what people *really* need or want in their final weeks, days, or hours. I met very few dying people concerned with heaven's blueprints, bodily resurrection, or lakes of fire. Instead, they wanted love, peace, and forgiveness. They depended upon hearing reassurances that God loved them and had forgiven them, and that their families loved and had forgiven them, too. They wanted to know that they would be remembered, and that the chaplain and the medical staff were doing all they could to ensure a peaceful and painless transition beyond the sick body they'd found themselves in.

We may believe that arming ourselves with all the scripture and doctrine in the world will help us conquer death, its fears, and its residual grief, but no one has the definitive religious or spiritual answers as to what happens to us when we die. As Nora told Mom and me that day in the church narthex—we don't *really* know, which leaves us with lots of questions. Faith, after all, is belief in that which we cannot see—nor completely know. For now, it's left to us to make sense and meaning out of the vocabulary we do have, even if we have to "flip the script," as Chaplain Sally told me.

"Open, open, open" (as I mentioned previously) was the mantra I clung to when I served patients. In dealing with my parents' deaths, I tried to imbibe that same grace for myself. I didn't know it all—and I *couldn't* know it all. Only, now, it was my parents who were on the other side of that thick curtain. I couldn't see through it nor move it, and it all felt so final. My finite human brain couldn't even compute all the possibilities.

So, I stuck with: *Open, open, open.*

I chose to be open to *every* possibility this side of heaven—even reincarnation.

"Is that you?" I began to inquire of every golden retriever, goat, grumpy senior, and old-souled toddler who resembled my dead loved ones.

"We *don't* know," Nora had said. "And that's the big question."

Chapter 6

Let's Talk about Death

"I realize how open we are to the persistent message that we can avert death. And to its punitive correlative, the message that if death catches us we have only ourselves to blame."
—Joan Didion, The Year of Magical Thinking

"Time is the school in which we learn,
Time is the fire in which we burn."
—Delmore Schwartz, *"Calmly We Walk through This April's Day,"* Summer Knowledge

The Grief Train

Grief, my therapist once told me, is a unique train ride in which the bereaved are often the sole passengers. It's a long journey through which we remember our loved ones, learn from the process, and receive moments of clarity about who we are without them. There is no fixed schedule, no pre-determined set of train cars, and no final destination. The train has no conductor—it just moves. There may be some useful, anticipated, or unanticipated visitors—former passengers on their own grief trains—who board along the way. We learn from their wisdom. Other times, the trip may seem isolated and purposeless. My therapist added that the train may even reverse directions, take an unexpected loop, slow its speed, or accelerate without warning. But it is *our* train, unique to each griever.

When my therapist first brought up this metaphor, I thought it to be the loneliest cross-country tour I'd ever heard of. Who wants to ride a damn imaginary train for an unknown amount of time in which there may or may not be a dining car with hot cocoa, restrooms, welcome visitors, or stops? *This ain't the Polar Express,* I thought.

Assuring me, she said it would all work out the way it was supposed to, because this was *my* train.

The stations, she said, were the points at which we receive clarity in our grief, processing the lessons gleaned from time spent in these "railroad cars": wisdom from former passengers who become mentors in our coping, as well as the support of our very-much-alive family and friends—all helpers and witnesses to our suffering.

"You are on your train right now," she told me, then added, "and remember, no two grief trains are alike."

There is no standard route in grief. As the wisest grievers I know have told me, "There is nowhere you can be but *in* it." There are, however, common "cars" we all ride in heartache—similar threads woven in the fabric of loss: first anniversaries, new years, meaning-making, identity struggles, emotional poles, struggles to talk about our grief and death itself, and—ultimately—*acceptance.* Those shared railcars serve as touchpoints of normalcy— connections through which we encounter wisdom and comfort in a mutual human experience. *Keep a look out for those cars and passengers,* my therapist said, *there you'll find the helpers, the mentors, and lessons that will unfurl.* These, she assured me, would help me discover my own stations: tools and meaning for my own path.

Station One: Time-Keeping

After my mother passed, I marked important days, events, and anniversaries by reading through old journal entries and listening to old voicemails, looking for glimpses of Mom to carry into the present.

On significant days such as my promotion to a new faculty position, her brother's death, the new book contract, a family reunion coordinated because I wanted her memory to live on—

these milestones served to both bring her close, but also to remind me she was gone. They reminded me I could no longer say, "Mom knew about this." Every day following August 24, 2017, was an inching further away from her knowing any of the events of my life.

Days marked on the calendar, hours on the clock, years marked with tears, pages written in the journal—are all integral to the bereaved.

Months after Mom died, I called her eldest brother's widow to invite her to that family reunion I organized. Uncle Charlie had been the first of my mother's five siblings to die—just four short years after their own mother's death. Though my aunt had been widowed nearly 20 years ago, she was the first to bring up her own grief train when I phoned.

As we talked she told me that, on one particular important grief anniversary, she woke up and just realized her husband wasn't coming back. "He ain't gonna come walkin' through that door ever again," she recounted to me as her thoughts from that time. "So, I said to myself, 'You can either stay miserable, or you can pick yourself up and get on with your life."

Listening to her talk provided me with the recognition of a daunting reality: I didn't want to pick myself up and get on with my life without my mother. But after we hung up, I realized I'd encountered a shared stop on the train, a brief moment of grief clarity. Though two decades had passed—and my uncle had existed *solely* in her (and our) memory for 20 years—my aunt's grief decisions—and her own train ride, seemed as fresh to her as Tuesday.

Grief never goes away, I realized. *It just changes shape.*

But finding fellow sojourners on the grief train who *understood* the way time-keeping and grief are inextricably linked felt like a rare gift.

In her memoir, *Everything Happens for a Reason: And Other Lies I've Loved,* Kate Bowler shares a courageous narrative of her Stage IV colon cancer diagnosis. At age 35 she was living her dream life: a tenure-track professor position at Duke, a perfect baby boy, and a strong marriage with her high-school sweetheart. And then her world exploded with one word: *cancer.*

"Ever since the diagnosis," she writes, "there has been a moment, in the minute between sleeping and waking, when I forget, when I have only a lingering sense that there is something I am supposed to remember."

Though describing what it feels like to *live* with a *terminal* diagnosis, Bowler's words precisely construct what the days and weeks following a loved one's death *also* feel like: that precious, dream-state moment every morning when the world—even if just for one breath—is whole again. It's the moment we've forgotten that our parent, our spouse, our best friend—or whoever our "person" might be—is gone. I woke up with this *exact* feeling every morning for six months after losing my mother.

Each morning, the alarm went off. And for those brief seconds before full awakening, I forgot I was still on the train.

"I used to think that grief was about looking backward," Bowler writes. "I see now that it is about eyes squinting through tears into an unbearable future." When death and dying arrive—whether swiftly, as in my father's cardiac arrest, or through a terminal diagnosis, as in my mother's perforated diverticulitis—future *time with them* vanishes. Every birthday, anniversary, family gathering, or circled calendar day that used to be previously anticipated—the joy, the laughs, the memories—lives under the fog of zero visibility. Time is ripped to shreds when you realize your loved one will not be there to share it with you.

You lose the ability to imagine the future will contain any morsel of happiness. Bowler describes being stuck in this kind of semi-permanent present tense. Some moments that first year, I found myself saying, *I can hold it together this minute, but the next minute is fair game.* This was especially true as I was forced to go about my regular routine, or "put on my clothes and act like I'm somebody," as my mother used to say. Mom also named and made personal this inability to anticipate and move oneself into the future, calling it, "My get up and go done got up and went."

Mom died the second week of my fall semester. As faculty, I couldn't simply push a pause button on my students' learning. I *had* to keep going. The grief train *had* to coincide with my daily teaching life, even if "my get up and go" was gone. There was an urgency to return to my courses, which, in some ways, was a welcome distraction. In other ways, it was a nightmare.

I remember distinctly one rainy commute to school. It was a September Wednesday after Mom's death, and I'd slinked out of bed to teach my 8:00 a.m. section of Critical Thinking. I was making a left-hand turn onto an on-ramp leading to our city's busiest beltline. Mid-turn, I asked myself, *How will I take this drive day after day, with no sense of the future, no faith or hope in this gut-level pain ending? How will I be able to stand this?*

Those first months, I *forced* myself from under the covers, but reserved commutes, bathroom breaks, solitary elevator rides, and rare moments alone in hallways and offices as opportunities to fall apart. I distinctly remember thinking: *How am I going to survive living minute to minute like this?*

Before her death, I saw Mom nearly daily, and spoke with her on the phone at several points throughout the day, including during that commute back and forth to school. After she died, these commutes—and the hours—felt empty. Where her voice had once been in my car, in my ear, and in my life, there was instead silence. I could no longer access her with a button, the ring of a phone.

The literal and metaphorical direct line I'd had to her for 36 years was cut off, without even notice first of a late bill. She just wasn't there. I tried to drown out the sadness with music or podcasts, but every lyric or lesson reminded me of her in some way—and, I would be right back where I had started: hours spent empty, lonely, and on a train I wanted to derail.

Loved ones told me this is often the hardest part of that first year: this inability to *plan* for a future with our loved ones—and the persistent absence of their voice. The loss of their bodily presence in a realm where we could see, touch, and hear them is so visceral you feel as if you're slowly bleeding to death, hour by hour.

Five months after my mother's August death, my grief train "hit a crossing." The train would not budge. The commuting tools that had helped me make it through the first holidays—Thanksgiving and Christmas—somehow left me unprepared for the New Year's arrival.

It was a new year. *Without mom.*

The proverbial calendar had flipped over, time had marched on, and the future had *arrived*, whether I liked it or not. I met a new phase of grief: determining what *meaning* Mom's death held for my new life without her.

Station Two: Meaning-Making

I found myself returning over and over to Joan Didion's wisdom in *The Year of Magical Thinking*, and Kate Bowler's willful prose on being terminal. I encountered them as sojourners—passengers on their own grief trains—who'd also taken the ride, and were now offering the wisdom of the shared cars, the journey, the long narrow tracks. They were part of the tribe of mentors who could assure me that the stations of clarity would arrive, and I was going to be OK.

From Didion I learned that "grief turns out to be a place none of us know until we reach it." We can make some generalizations, certainly, about the train ride everyone takes: from the initial shock, to the five stages Elisabeth Kübler-Ross so famously outlined in her book, *On Death and Dying*.

But the day-to-day grip of filling the void eludes us. "Only the survivors of death are truly left alone," Didion concludes. "The connections that made up their life...have all vanished."

Mom had vanished. The woman I used to visit and speak with every day of my life was gone.

Living the routines and rituals that once involved our loved ones are difficult enough. Memory "vortexes," as Didion calls them, can feel even worse, because they appear out of nowhere, even as the brain and body believe they are *purposefully* avoiding thinking of the deceased. Vortexes are those innocuous thoughts that lead to other seemingly innocuous thoughts, until you arrive at a germ of a memory of your loved one. "The way you got side-swiped," wrote Didion, "was by going back."

I didn't want to go back to memories of her—it was too painful—but neglecting the loss...was *worse*. I needed those reels of Mom to remind me that she'd lived, and help me understand why the grief felt so real and raw. I needed them to discover how I'd make sense and meaning out of all this hurt.

Vivid dreams were common cars on my grief train. I wrote each dream down, desperate to grip fleeting dawn details, hopeful for clues they'd left me. I hoped for signposts to signal a new lesson, provide some clarity—or, better yet, a message that the trip was coming to a close, and soon I could exit, leave the train's journey, and say, "Well, thank God *that's* over."

But there is no full-on end to the loss, no final destination in grief. No leaving the train.

I had recurring dreams about my paternal Grandmother Dorothy, who died my second year of seminary. In one dream, I rummaged through the familiar dresser drawers in the one-story Indiana retirees' apartment she shared with my grandfather. In the dream, her bedroom is intact; the furniture and its contents haven't been moved, and I know what's in each drawer, since I'd seen her open them thousands of times. As I spread my hands over her belongings, I'm not certain what it is I'm looking for. Jewelry is my best guess, as we both shared a passion for all things shiny and tacky.

When I shared this dream with chaplain friends, they told me I wasn't looking for material goods of Grandmother's at all; I was looking for the "gold": the *valuable meaning* amid the loss.

I began to learn to read the grief dreams on the train and to anticipate other signs for meaning—some that arrived even during the waking hours.

For example, nearly eight months after my mother died, I opened her Bible for the first time. A piece of paper clipped to the first page had an undated handwritten note that read:

"Forgive me.

I forgive you.

Thank you.

I love you.

Goodbye.

My final words before passing."

It came special delivery, an undated grief parcel of meaning. I was just *certain* it hadn't been there before—after all, we'd had her Bible and everything from her hospice bedside—and had never noticed it paper-clipped to the inside. I wondered if she'd sent it after her death, a reassurance that we'd said what we'd needed to say, and that the labor of Mom's death had been sufficient.

Didion writes that death and grief are full of symbols and omens that yield meaning. Did my mother know I would need that note? Had she sent it *after* her death? Did the founder of the now-ubiquitous Death Café movement know that following its advent he was going to die? Was it inclination—or, a strange force drawing him to do the work of wrestling with death, to be ready for his own?

Years ago, I thought of writing a book similar to this one. I'd survived hospital chaplaincy, my father's death, and Fred's father's death. During a family gathering, I sat in our apartment living room with my husband, mom, and in-laws, and told them I was scared to write down all I'd learned in chaplaincy from the dying: I feared it would bring about someone's death.

Three years later, in August 2017, my mother died.

On the "train," Didion taught me that survivors *do* see—or, at least, they read meaning into what they perceive to be messages they missed. The bereaved, she wrote, "live by symbols," adding connotation to the seemingly mundane.

Station Three: Identity

Following Mom's death, I spent 13 months in hospice grief counseling, scrambling to find new tools and work harder for the lessons—the stations of clarity that I wanted to arrive at quicker and move through faster. I wanted to get grief "done"—like a to-do list—and deboard this damn train. That first year, I attended grief workshops and kept a detailed grief notebook. I made terrible art projects out of clay and paint. I strapped Mom's ashes in my passenger seat and took her on road trips. I *planted* myself neck deep in my mother's death in those first few months as I ticked off the tasks—for, I couldn't see a future without her. I couldn't see myself.

Is this, I ask, what grief *feels* like: a desperate need to discover meaning amid a loss of self, a rupture of our identity, a sudden void—a disappearance of those who have shaped and formed us? Are lost loved ones the start of an ongoing quest to find meaning *and* discover who we are on the other side of loss? Who we are without our parents or grandparents? Who we are without our partners? Without our best friends? Who are we if we are not someone's granddaughter, daughter, or wife? These relationships help define us, and their sudden loss is suffocating, because we do not know who we are anymore.

When someone close dies, the ripe, plump fullness we knew ourselves to be, as seen in and among those who have lived alongside us, knowing our stories—many since our births—is simply gone.

At one session of hospice grief counseling, I stormed in, talking a mile a minute and asking all these questions. I'd built up an arsenal of things that needed to be processed. I told my counselor about this swirl of conflicting emotions and identity crises. Some moments, when I tried to make meaning out of what was happening, the sadness for Mom being gone felt like too much, like I—my identity—was going to get stuck in the abyss of grief and I would never scratch my way out.

Those were the hours I missed her so viscerally I could vomit. But other hours I felt so free for her and me that I sang my favorite songs at inappropriate volume because I felt relief for us both.

I can still picture the *look* on the hospice counselor's face that day as my words rushed out at her. Without speaking, she simply took a deep breath. I mirrored her instantly, as she knew I would.

"OK. You know you don't need to figure all this out *right* now," she'd said.

And yet I longed to read meaning into every mood, moment, and memory—to let myself be sad, but I was floundering to understand the moments I felt relief in my newfound identity without her.

The hospice counselor assured me that this was "spot on." I was *not* losing my mind. I was *actually* grieving. And, as with processing *any* big life event or relationship change, the hours were dynamic. Some minutes would *feel* like two contradictory emotional ends of a pole, and that was normal.

I'd never had these emotional poles with the loss of anyone else, because my identity had not ever been so enmeshed with anyone else. This was the difference between grieving my mother and grieving my father. Mom was my source and mirror—a significant part of what I thought made me *me*. When she died, I had time and ability to process who I was without her. Dad, on the other hand, had been distant all my life, like a satellite dimly broadcasting a fuzzy picture. When he died a month before my wedding, the letter had been sent, he'd already been cut off, and there was no time to dissect meaning and identity. There were wedding details to organize, a man to marry, and a mother to take care of. I took *no time* to grieve.

Now, I was swinging the other way, taking a bit *too much time* to think about it all at once—trying to *control* a train I couldn't conduct, *over-processing* who I was amid loss, chastising myself that I wasn't mourning 24/7...and horrified at the times when I was.

I wanted to *feel* my grief *deeply* and figure out who I am as a result of it. But my counselor reminded me that it was also OK to have hours "off" from all this searching. I needed to take deep breaths, gaze out the grief train's window, and remember there was still a living world of focus and function, and singing and laughter. It was all OK, because it was *my* grief train.

Grief, my hospice counselor taught me, was about offering ourselves radical grace and self-care while encountering all these emotions, questions, and experiences on the train. We ride in railcars of deep despair and relief—and even *euphoria* that our loved one isn't suffering or in pain, that they are in peace and not enduring endless surgeries, treatments, or medicines to repair an aging body that cannot be fixed. But there are also cars of identity—for determining who we are as we navigate the world without our people.

Being kind to myself while sitting in all these *different* railroad car seats was important. I needed to hold the sorrow *and* reprieve, acknowledging the immense gratitude I felt for her suffering to have ended. It was OK to despair *and* be joyful at the same time. It was OK to search for myself. This was the journey. I wasn't expected to sit in the *very same* seat for the entire ride.

But I couldn't have known all this was normal unless I had been willing to *talk* with others about it, and they had been willing to *talk* with me, too.

Station Four: Talking about Grieving

Intellectually, I "knew" death and grief. As a minister and chaplain, I'd read books, learned the stages, and cared for the dying and bereaved.

But I belong to a culture that tucks death away in hospitals and nursing homes, that banishes grief with clever social media posts that ward off reality. So, how is it possible to begin to broach the taboo topic of mourning a loss when so few people are willing to even acknowledge its existence?

Bystanders generally believe that—outside traditional, private counseling settings—the bereaved don't want to *talk* about grief, hear about, or speak of the dead. But one of the most comforting things is for someone to utter our loved one's *name*, or lend an ear—even if both are offered only briefly. A memory lifted or a simple, "I miss her, and know you do, too," is a significant touchpoint. While others cannot ride your grief train for you, to know that they *see* you—this is comforting. They know *where* you are, and what it *feels* like to be there—perhaps because they've been there themselves. They understand what it means to love and lose.

Without those touchpoints—the grief "crutches" of train car passengers' support that came in the form of coffee with best friends, phone calls, cards, and lessons from Didion, Bowler, Kübler-Ross, and fellow chaplains—I would not have survived. I would not have grieved Mom well—and, I'm not certain what would have happened to me. My best guess is that I'd still be at that left turn at the on-ramp, unable to envision any future, any hope, and wondering, *How will I make it through?*

From the ridiculous airline safety videos, to American culture's obsessive fear of aging and our avoidance of death, we just don't want to acknowledge or talk about "it"—grief, death, dying...*any* of it. And for the grieving, this can be devastating.

Of all the people I've met over the years, very few understood all the train cars running the grief tracks: time-keeping, meaning-making, identity, emotional poles, and the importance of naming the reality of loss. Those who understood—my mother, fellow chaplains, pastors, ministers, counselors, and others—were those who'd grieved *deeply,* and had helped others do the same. Most everyone else I encountered seemed oblivious to the fact that people just *dropped dead* and left others behind to mourn them. Of course, it wasn't *their* fault they couldn't name the obvious. It was just *American.* This culture isn't exactly known for its profound chats on mortality. Weather and scandalous reality TV show characters, yes. Dying, no.

During that year of ministering in the hospital, we learned what one minister friend aptly named the "chaplain's sacred walk of death." That is, we learned that unique perspective chaplains are privy to in partially entering into the *other* side of the curtain—the *real* side of life (death and subsequent grief). It's the behind-the-curtain experience my mother thought of when she drafted her advance directives papers in 1997, telling Ron and me exactly how she wanted to die. The "sacred walk of death" is life's *heartache,* the reality of taking care of and *being* with people who are finishing up "their assignments" here on earth, as I once heard a wise spiritual woman call them. Chaplain residency taught me how to walk with patients in their final days, hours, and moments, we learned the many gifts of leaving—including a clarity of what's important—and gained the ability to *talk* to others about the important lessons we'd received from the sacred walk of death.

After my mother's death, I had a small, core group of friends who became frequent companions on my grief train. They were the first to acknowledge that the ride is not a ticket anybody wants. They understood when I spoke of the train's speed, its overwhelming—and sometimes *underwhelming*—pace. These friends reassured me that despite twists and turns, lulls and lags, acceleration and whiplash, there's nowhere you can be but in it.

We'd often commiserate about why few people can—or want to—acknowledge the heaviness of grief, a fact that is so integral to life. We talked for hours long-distance about this mystery. Their willingness to talk about grief made the ride bearable.

Rev. Sally Bates was one of those consistent conversation partners on the train. From time to time, we'd meet to talk about my mother's death and subsequent grief trains we'd encountered—including those of her family and friends. When she cared for a friend during the last days in ICU, she was, like me, appalled at the way Americans erase death—and its aftermath—from Main Street. "We've banished both birth and death from our households, bedrooms, and parlors," she said, "and sent it off to the sterile land of modern medicine."

Comparing notes on ICU pastoral care, we talked about how raw and *real* death is in those hospital units, and how strange life feels when you step outside into a world that pretends as if mourning isn't a thing—or, at the very least, it's something to overcome, and *quickly*. Even though it's normal, and all of us *will* experience it, our skittishness about life's end isn't useful when it comes time to process the grief.

It wasn't until Mom's death, and with the gift of those ongoing conversations with Sally and others, that I *intentionally* began to wrestle with how close grief had hit home—and just how meaningful a part of my life it had become.

If my fate was to ride this grief train, I wanted to *understand* it so I could help others understand it, too. Moments of literal and metaphorical "tea and coffee" with fellow sojourners were an important part of that. Sally and friends kept me an active participant in my own grieving, by *talking* about it, so that I could make sense of it for myself. To *talk* about grief is to *make* it a part of living.

But we *don't want to* talk about grief. We fear being "Debbie Downer," the exaggerated *Saturday Night Live* character who disrupts bowling night with her gutter balls of reality. But culture and conversation *will have to* shift to being more open soon, out of necessity. The number of dying Americans is expected to rise by more than one-third in the next 20 years, thanks to the Baby Boomers. The Baby Boomers—the generation to which my father belonged—is the largest *living* generation, and they will soon be the largest *dying* generation. Like my father—who was born in 1946—the Boomers have lessons for us, even as we (and they) may do our best to ensure that death, grief, and all related questions are still hidden under the table. With the death tsunami coming, more of us will be riding grief trains, so we need to start the larger, public conversation.

An unwillingness to acknowledge reality has grave consequences. For those hovering between a good quality of life and their final years, weeks, or days—*not* talking about *death*—from brass tacks to big, meaningful things that *need* to be said, can be devastating.

I learned this from another sojourner who arrived in my life *prior* to Mom's death, but whose wisdom echoed as I rode my own grief train. Rev. Stimpson "Stimp" Hawkins, retired Presbyterian minister, had a long career in pastoring and hospice chaplaincy. In those years he'd known birth and death: he'd seen relationships blossom and decay, children succeed and disappoint, faith grow and doubt crush. Stimp, along with my mother, showed me that these losses clarify yet another station on the grief train: *anticipating* and *preparing* for death.

Station 5: Talking about Death

Stimp was a part of the "The Positive Death Movement"— positive in that it doesn't view death as a shameful, taboo topic. Like Mom, he was a part of a relatively small set of the population: older adults who actively talk about and plan for death. Few Americans give death consistent public air time, but

"The Positive Death Movement" is a growing one, brought on in part by the Baby Boomers. Evidence of its growth is visible in "The Conversation Project," Death Cafés, Death Doulas, the "Ask a Mortician" YouTube series, and best-selling books on death and dying. It offers a constructive approach to mortality.

I was introduced to "Stimp, the Death Pimp," as he was known in central North Carolina, while attending a Buddhist Meditation Center. He was the wisest, mellowest octogenarian I'd ever met. In the short time I knew him, Stimp changed my understanding of how we all *could* approach death—whether we are 82 or 18.

Stimp earned his moniker through participating and serving as a facilitator, teacher, and willing participant in any setting in which folks needed a little nudge on how to start "the conversation." He spent his final years ensuring that everyone he encountered *knew* that they had more control over their death than they realized—all they had to do was *talk about it.*

Planning for our own deaths, he said, is the "greatest gift" we could ever give ourselves and our loved ones.

"All we have is this moment," Stimp always said as he patted his shirt pocket where he kept his M.O.S.T. (Medical Orders for Scope of Treatment) papers with him 24/7.

"Should I fall out right here, y'all know what to do—or rather, what not to do," he added, in his Virginian accent. Stimp, at 82, was so fervent in his wishes for a peaceful passing of *only* comfort care that, not only had he prepared all the *legal* papers to reflect his wishes, but he also had had "D.N.R." (Do Not Resuscitate) tattooed above his heart—with a monkey underneath. The tattoo ink, of course, offered no legal weight, but served as a symbol and reminder to reinforce the legal ink he'd placed on paper: his declaration of intent for a natural death.

Stimp's "Death Pimp" ways of "Let's Talk about Death" galvanized conversation—and action. It also garnered statewide attention. WUNC, our NPR affiliate, interviewed him *live* during his own cardboard-casket signing party.

"I want to die *naturally*," Stimp told Frank Stasio, North Carolina host of the radio show *The State of Things*. "I've had a great life. When it's my turn to go, I'm ready." Stimp had indeed had a wonderful life: four children, one stepdaughter, and 12 grandchildren who adored him. He spread his mantra of *"JOY!"* (his favorite word) everywhere he went. Stimp had *charisma*; a true minister and chaplain, within minutes of meeting you, he could get almost *anyone* to open up about *everything*—from sharing your life story to unwittingly sharing how you wanted to die.

No one could resist Stimp's charm—evidenced by the fact that he even convinced Stasio to get *inside and lay down* in Stimp's casket on stage during a live broadcast. Stimp was ready for death, and wanted everyone else to *feel* a bit readier, too. The death conversation was one he was passionate about, and he helped others voice it—openly, honestly, with care *and* humor.

Nearly six months to the day after Stasio interviewed him, Stimp died. Stimp's widow, Dr. Martha Taylor—a registered licensed dietician, professor, and hospice consultant—now continues to champion Stimp's mission to educate others on death. Martha and Stimp were regulars at Greensboro's Death Café and Café Mortale, where Stimp would lead with the obvious conversation starter: *always* be prepared to die.

Stimp believed people were hesitant to talk about death because of the unknown. No one knows exactly what the afterlife will be like. Denial, Stimp felt, is a powerful sentiment. By having death conversations, Stimp believed, and in discussing our death wishes and plans, we take away the *power* of its sting. The grief train, in turn, becomes easier to ride.

His number one rule was: Start the conversation. "None of us is getting out of here alive," he'd say, laughing. The conversation, he insisted, "is the biggest gift you can give your family."

Stimp's insistence on talking about death ensured his family's grief train would already be on the tracks—equipped with tools his loved ones needed to remember and mourn him well. He knew the train was unavoidable, so packing for the ride was key. How could he prepare them to make the ride—even in its sorrow— more comfortable?

He *reminded* them he was going to die—we *all* are. He talked about death. He lessened their fears by showing his courage in facing the inevitable. Stimp planned his own memorial service, secured his casket, got the casket signed by friends and family, and even ensured that there would be handwritten notes of encouragement for his loved ones to revisit when they needed company and assurance on their grief train.

No detail had been left undone. All this *talking* about death— these arrangements and assurances—freed his family and friends to be in their grief, to simply *remember* their beloved father, grandfather, friend, and mentor well.

Stimp died according to his plan—at home with hospice. Martha and his children engaged in his care. When the time drew near, the funeral home brought the signed cardboard casket—the one he *and* Frank Stasio had lain in on stage. Finally, Stimp was placed inside, sent off with a Bible verse and love.

That first, innocuous meeting at the Buddhist Center unfurled into hours of conversation about death. Stimp, Martha, Fred, and I kept in close touch. In just a few years of knowing him, Stimp offered me lessons I didn't know I'd need so badly—ones that would continue to remain with me during Mom's death, and on my own grief ride.

Station Six: Acceptance

A few years before Mom died, I led a writing retreat at which I met a fellow Baptist who specializes in grief care. Rev. Brad Mitchell is an ordained pastor and grief counselor who works closely with a funeral home in his community.

Since I'd found so few people who *understood* the grief train—who actively wanted to talk about the stations of grief and death—I reached out to Brad after Mom died. I imagined him as part of a group of "morbid grief train superheroes," who I'd secretly dubbed "The Death Squad." Sally was among this crew, as are Joan Didion and Kate Bowler. During my grief train journey, I considered them welcome companions—safe people whose wisdom I could dive into deeply and quickly.

Brad is a gracious member of "The Death Squad," confirmed by his willingness to talk about his end-of-life doctoral work in pastoral care, as well as his professional and personal experience with assisting others on their own grief trains. He is someone who *sees* and processes death *every* day in his work as a pastor, grief counselor, and community partner for his local funeral home. And among his gifts to me was the way in which he entertained my ongoing, nagging question: "If this is something we *all* go through, why do we avoid talking about it?"

"Unknowns bring fear," he responded, corroborating Stimp's experience. "Most people will avoid anything that brings them fear." Grief is frightening, and death is, too. This understandably makes people anxious, he explained.

When I asked how he—as Stimp could—got people to open up amid fear, and talk about their grief and death, he reiterated what every chaplain, minister, and dying person I've ever met has shown me: *presence*. Presence means we are willing to accept the uncomfortable circumstance over which we have no control in order to *sit with it*. Whether in grief, difficult conversations about end-of-life, or actual times of death, there's nothing more required of us than to just be in it.

But why is it so *hard*?

Brad suggested that it's because we don't practice. We don't accept it, in order to just *be*. We get nervous, dance around these tough topics, and try to fix them. Our unwillingness to sit with the hard stuff leads to harmful, hurtful, and insensitive sentiments—even when they are meant from a place of love and care.

Similar to Kate Bowler, Brad offered me specifics of how to be present, instead of saying those "what *not to say*" comments when grief or death come up in conversation. What are those unhelpful comments? Brad nominated phrases such as: "They lived a long life—you should be grateful;" "They are in a better place;" "Heaven gained an angel;" and, "God needed them more than we do."

Acceptance that leads into our *being present,* in Brad's experience, is far better when words fail us and we want to solve the unsolvable or skirt the unavoidable for fear of the unknown. Often, our *presence*—not our Pollyanna responses—is what is needed most.

Brad also reminded me that *each person's* perception of death, dying, and grief is different. We are all on our own grief trains; we talk about, face, and cope with death and grieve *differently*. From my brother Ron, to me, to Fred, to my aunt, to Sally, to Stimp and Martha—we have our own tracks. There are common threads—time-keeping, meaning-making, identity struggles, and stations of clarity. But our direct experience is unique to us. Brad reminded me that grief expectations and timelines imposed on others are not useful. In beautiful candor about processing his own father's death, he admitted to me that he preferred to grieve *alone*.

When he said this, he didn't realize the gift he'd given me. I'd struggled with the fact that I often didn't want to express public emotion over my mother's death. I let very few people onto the train with me. Some of this I attributed to the cultural and societal norms around grieving, but some of it felt like personal preference (though, I did blubber like a baby during her *entire* funeral).

Grieving alone, Brad added, meant that people didn't experience him grieving as they might have expected. After his father died, he grieved in unconventional ways: jogging and writing. He always held his composure in public—until a year after his father's death.

He was at a ceremony to which he had been invited, during which his deceased father's memory was honored. At the event, Brad was overcome with grief. Unable to push down tears, he showed his emotion and cried in public. When a family member told him that she was "glad to see you finally let it go," it sparked his frustration with the lack of understanding that comes from that kind of comment—a frustration he relayed to me: "I hadn't met her expectations, so she had missed the fact that I had adequately grieved in other ways," Brad said. "We have to be careful not to project our own way of grieving onto others—it's a weight they do not wish to bear."

Grief—I realized again—dissolves, changes form. We might move to another railroad car on the train and find a change of scene; maybe this car has fresher air, with a view of soothing landscapes enjoyed from brighter seats.

Mom's sudden illness and death brought about an urgency to talk about grief and death, but I had to do it my own way. I needed my own "Death Squad"—those mentors along the way whose wisdom brought moments of clarity when the train slowed into a station and the sun shone bright through the windows.

I knew that at some point on the journey, my itinerary would shift. I would need to share the lessons I learned—the waves, the loops, the permission to grieve, the coaches, and the meaning-making—with others. As we march toward the upcoming "big death tsunami" of the Boomers, we must face the looming reality with tools—beginning with how we talk about, understand, and accept the single most *certain* aspect of life: death.

Once we understand the grief train, and talk about it, we can talk about our own deaths.

Chapter 7

Beginning with the End in Mind

"Is it possible to befriend our dying...to prepare for our death with the same attentiveness that our parents had in preparing for our birth?"
—Henri Nouwen, Our Greatest Gift: A Meditation on Dying and Caring

Be Prepared

Nearly all of us have encountered the scout motto, "Be prepared." But, "prepared" for *what?* Getting lost in the woods? Building shelter? Mending split pants? Hustling a hungry passerby into buying cookies and popcorn?

My mother didn't know her way around a Swiss Army knife, but she knew that, at its core, the scout motto had less to do with saving one's own neck than with *helping* others. She embraced the mantra, "Be prepared," in living—and in dying—because she knew it would help her two children when the day came. Two decades before she passed away, Mom had already told me and Ron *exactly* how she wanted to die.

She had legal advance directives drawn up in 1997—in black-and-white, and notarized. I was only 16; Ron was 34; she was 57.

The paperwork (her living will) declared her desire for a natural death and gave Ron her health-care power of attorney. When she *did* become terminally ill, her line of thinking—planning in advance for death—was still considered an anomaly among society in general, just like Stimp's. Among her octogenarian peers at the assisted living facility where she spent her last seven months, she was known as the "youngster" (being still shy of 80). So nearly everyone—from her fellow residents to staff to her doctors—was puzzled as to why a seemingly healthy 70-something *wanted* to be prepared for dying.

Three years prior to her death, her primary care physician *finally* agreed it was appropriate to sign her "golden pages" Do-Not-Resuscitate Order. She brought the document home and taped it to the refrigerator with great pride, amid photos of the grandkids held by magnets of her favorite cities.

The Christmas before her death, she outlined her own memorial service in a red spiral notebook, complete with eulogy themes, hymn choices, and even the specific day of the week and time she wanted it to occur.

This was all completed by a woman who, at the time, was not terminally ill. She didn't have cancer or a chronic disease that would wipe her out at any second—she just *knew* what she wanted. She wanted to "be prepared."

Much of mom's death planning stemmed from having been on the "other side of the curtain," as she called it. She had been a nurse for well over 30 years, a medical professional who *saw* what could happen if you hadn't made decisions—or had failed to tell your family about those decisions—in advance. Mom had witnessed firsthand the effects *not* talking about death had had on her patients and their families. That's why she made her wishes *abundantly* clear to me and Ron, and made us promise that we would honor (and enforce) them under any circumstance.

Even within her field of medicine, her preparations made her an outlier. With *no* hint that death was imminent, she'd taken the time two decades ago to legally document her wishes. Then, when she was diagnosed with a life-threatening sudden illness, she perplexed her doctors—since they couldn't imagine a relatively healthy woman saying "No!" to a straightforward, feasible surgery to repair a perforated intestine. For that also meant she was saying no to a surgery that would keep her from *dying*. But for Mom, the diverticulitis had perforated her intestines for a *reason,* and fixing it surgically went against two of her core values: first, her "no knives" policy, and second, prolonging the inevitable, natural process already underway in her infected body.

The night Mom was admitted to the hospital, Ron immediately extinguished eager surgeons' wishes to fix the problem. He requested that they *only* stabilize her, and pitch the ball to a non-curative, palliative care team as soon as they could. Reluctantly they did so.

With a clear set of her wishes, we had a firm plan in place. Ron used his medical expertise to outline her plan of care and execute next steps: he asked surgeons and all hospital doctors assigned to Mom to administer *only* enough curative treatment to stabilize Mom enough for me to return home from my business trip, and for her to comfortably enjoy a long weekend "party" of goodbyes with her family. Then she was to be transitioned to comfort care at hospice as soon as possible.

Mom—alert, awake, and with her wits about her the entire time she was hospitalized—affirmed these as her wishes. She was proud that we understood and implemented her plan. We did so only because, for decades, she'd lived by her "be prepared" motto, and now it was time to die by it.

"It's a great life if you don't weaken," Mom used to say. To her, a life was made meaningful by *facing* tough issues with strength.

The "D Word"

Whether because we view it as un-American, or consider it to foreshadow a "Grim Reaper" tea party, most of us would rather die than *talk* about dying. The English language uses hundreds of euphemisms for death for this very reason—because we'd rather not even utter the "D Word."

Had he been alive to hear Mom's story, Stimp would have approved of Mom's embrace of the "D Word." They both taught me that, in as much as we can "control" various aspects of our death, we should—and get to planning our "good death" *now.* Of course, there were things we'd *never know, nor be able to control,* about death: not when it comes, nor necessarily what will be the precipitating factors. But they both would have said, with a smile, we can "be prepared." It may be a simple 15-minute family meeting at Thanksgiving—or legal, official forms—but these plans are the "gift" we give ourselves, our loved ones, and anyone caring for us at the end of life. Stimp encouraged me to embrace *my own* plan for death— even in my 30s. Others think that's scary, crazy, or eerily ominous. But for me, what's more frightening and daunting is complete *silence* around a person's wishes, because I've *seen* its implications with my own eyes. I've sat through hours of meetings in hospital family rooms, comforting relatives torn apart over decisions they must make regarding their comatose loved one's care. When no one knows our wishes, and the unthinkable happens, devastating situations arise that could have otherwise been avoided.

While we are invited to respect every person's process—and understand that, like each unique grief train, everyone has both shared *and* unique experiences—my mother taught me that *ignoring* death doesn't lift anyone's burdens *when* the time does come. Mom thought it selfish to believe that others can or should handle difficult life decisions amid a stressful medical crisis. As with Stimp's ministry career, my mother's nursing career allowed her to witness many life-altering medical emergencies, and she believed that not discussing them in advance—especially when it concerned older adults—put undue stress on everyone. The strain, she said, was completely preventable, if people would just be willing to *start* a conversation about planning to be prepared for the "what ifs."

I don't think any of us really *wants* to die—unless, maybe if Al Roker and the *Today Show* have already framed your face inside that Smucker's "Happy Birthday!" label 10 times. When you're 110, physically suffering, and nearly everyone you know is already dead—then, yes, you may *want* to "bite the dust" or "enter the Pearly Gates."

We prepare extensively for births and adoptions: we "shower" expectant and adoptive mothers with all they will need to feed, clothe, and shelter their babies. Doctors, nurses, midwives, and doulas care for pregnant women—ensuring that mother and baby are healthy, and that the birth is safe. Our partners join us for hours of Lamaze class; we read *What to Expect When You Are Expecting*. We prepare nurseries, paint children's rooms, and hire attorneys to finalize adoptions. We invest *a lot* of time in these "birth" processes, no matter their details.

But with very little preparation, 2,712,630 people died in 2015 in the United States, or around 7,400 people per day. Hardly any of us have any paperwork ready, nor have we even considered talking with our families about how we want to die—or about what happens next.

Every *other* life milestone we have requires an *investment* of time to do it right—whether it is K-12 education, GED completion, community college, giving birth, adopting a child, getting married, vocational training, or simply on-the-job learning.

Until I literally *saw* my first death as a chaplain—Lily—I was struck by how little I'd thought about my own death. I hadn't made any plans, nor invested any time in understanding dying and what I wanted—and Lily and I had been nearly the same age.

Beginning with the End in Mind

When our great-great-great-great-great-grandrelatives died, they died at home. Our families cared for them when they became ill. They did their best to keep them warm, dry, safe, and comforted. Preachers may have been called to be bedside; prayers may have been said. Their bodies were cleaned and prepared for burial—usually in a church graveyard or family cemetery, if they had one.

Back then, there was no booming funeral industry. We didn't need papers to know so much about all the intricacies of what we—or loved ones—would need at the end of life. People simply got sick, old, or hurt—and they *died*. There was no readily available, aggressive, curative treatments and ambulances to transport them to facilities that could extend their lives—or at least slow their deaths—outside the family home. These weren't really decisions to be made; nature simply took its course.

Today's endless possibilities of medical interventions require we give careful thought to our preferences and wishes. Should we happen to suffer a horrible accident, endure a traumatic brain injury, lose function of several limbs, and be placed on life support, what level of care would we want, if any?

With so many curative treatments, we are invited to parse the options, and to ensure that someone knows our wishes in order to advocate for us should we not be able to do so for ourselves. Prior to Lily, chaplaincy, and—eventually—Mom's death, none of this truly sank in with me. But after Lily, I saw the *same* scene over and over on replay: patient suffers medical catastrophe, patient is terminal and unable to speak for themselves, patient's family is forced to make heart-wrenching decisions. Each catastrophe was different in its details, but the outcome was always the same: the patient was going to die, and there were threads that they—and their loved ones—could have anticipated prior to arriving to the Emergency Department. But because they were scared of the "D Word," they failed to begin with the end in mind.

Mom used those death papers she signed and kept safe in her filing cabinet to teach Ron and me how she wanted to die. Sometimes, it was through an obvious conversation, like the first time she said, "Here are my papers"; other times, it was subtler. But all of it led to those last two weeks of her life, when—though there were many *unknowns* about her body's unique shut-down process—there were many *knowns* we could be certain of. This knowledge made our remaining time with her more precious— as well as giving us more time with her, rather than needing to spend it chasing down or creating paperwork.

Because our mother began with the end in mind, she covered all the possible decisions we'd have to make, so that our only job was to *be present with her* as she faced death.

Following are some of the decisions she talked with us about— often over slow meals that began with her favorite dessert.

Before Death: Don't Take Your Organs to Heaven

Mom joked that she always wanted her body "donated to science," believing her body, after death, could at least be offered as an educational tool for research. As it turns out, this process is more complicated than it sounds. And while she was unable ultimately to donate her body to science, she ensured that everyone—including us—*learned* from the example of her wishes.

When I was teenager, Mom took me to a family doctor who drove an old, beat-up, hunter-green truck with a bumper sticker that read:

"Don't take your organs with you to heaven. Heaven knows we need them here."

Though I saw that bumper sticker many, *many* times, it didn't mean much to me until my mother took me to get my license at age 16. I never considered whether I wanted to be an organ donor until the DMV asked me if I wanted the red heart emoji on my driver's license.

Later, as a chaplain, I *saw* the urgent need for vital organs, and the life-saving role they play for children and adults who have complex medical emergencies and needs.

I also learned quickly that organ donation is far more nuanced than its Hollywood portrayals. Our stereotype is that scrubbed surgeons are waiting by ER doors for ambulances so they can open patients' wallets and look for heart emojis. We imagine that the heart gives them the green light to *immediately* divvy up our organs into YETI coolers that will hop the next flight to Phoenix. This is *not* at all how it works. Organ donation is a complex, intricate, careful process in which *everyone*—including our families—must be on board. And it's worth the time it takes to research our wishes.

When I got my first driver's license, Mom had already ensured that I knew about—and had thought about—what that heart icon meant. "It is your decision," she counseled. But what she did insist on is that I carefully consider the issue as a part of the privilege of earning a license. I could say no to organ donation, she said, but she wanted me to be fully aware of the options.

Before Death: Wills and Estates

Mom updated her will several times in her life. She taught us it was the responsibility of adults to determine how bank accounts, personal property, assets, and money were distributed after death. What person/people, organization, church, or charity would we like to bequeath those funds and/or property to? Without a legal will, our estate and affairs become the government's concern, and the situation becomes far more complex, depending upon your state's laws.

A few years prior to her death, Mom took me to her bank and added me to all her accounts. Our mother insisted the power over financial decisions and assets always reside within the family. As Mom would say, she "barely had a pot to pee in," but she always had her papers in order.

Before Death: Ashes to Ashes, or Six Feet Under?

Our mother was crystal clear about her wishes for cremation. She'd chosen it because it was economical and practical. The cemetery where she would have liked to have been buried had no plots remaining near to her parents, and her family's cemetery had long since become overgrown and wasn't easily accessible. Her considerate decision freed me, Ron, and Fred from having to scramble to find another burial plot—and it has made for fantastic stories and road trips with her Sunset Scatter box. Who would have ever thought we'd get so much mileage (literally) out of our mother's remains? We've laughed and cried over them. I've held her like an infant on days when I needed her close by. Cremation has allowed Mom to be *both* with us and *in* her favorite places (including the beach) simultaneously.

The only request we didn't honor (and now I wish we had), was the removal of her gold teeth to be made into jewelry.

After Mom was cremated, Sally and I joked about how the funeral industry has *everything*, literally, to commemorate the dead—from fingerprint jewelry to dissolving sand dollars made of loved ones' ashes. Sally's father was cremated and scattered (well, *dumped*, urn and all) at sea during a storm—after her mother became sea sick and yelled, "Just throw him overboard!" Later, her *mother's* cremated remains were mistaken at airport security for a *canned ham*.

"She would have had to have been a *smoked* ham," Sally added, because she, like my mother, appreciated the absurdity of it all.

"Urns, hand-crafted boxes, mantelpiece clocks and statuary, fine gemstone jewelry—you can literally get *anything*," she told me. When her friend died just a day after July 4, she added, "His family said, 'Well, we could have packed him in a firecracker and shot him into space.'"

Beginning with *The Big Lebowski*, to the urn scene in *Meet the Parents*, and followed by the ashes-in-a-coffee-can episode from *Due Date*, the cremation industry bears the brunt of mishaps regarding human remains. But Mom was very clear that she wanted to be scattered at the beach—windy day or not—and we honored that request, and added quite a few other destinations of which she would have approved. There are, of course, legal considerations with either option—cremation *or* burial. We should avoid burying our loved ones in the middle of the town square on a whim with a shovel; we should also avoid dumping five pounds of Grandpa's ashes into his enemy's well. Mom believed in employing advance conversation tactics (with humor!) to help us know her wishes—and ours—so we can secure what works legally and best for everyone.

During Death: Hospital Resources and Rituals

Because I'd been a chaplain, Mom had been keen on pastoral care services. So one of the first phone calls I made when she was admitted to the intensive care unit was to request this support. I knew a chaplain's presence would be comforting to her and Ron until I could catch a flight home.

Chaplains are the go-to resources for families caring for loved ones. During Mom's time at both the hospital and at hospice, chaplains were our mainstay. They know what is available for families. Like spiritual social workers, they can point us in the right direction, and match us with appropriate resources for our situations.

When I worked in the hospital as a chaplain, I appreciated the collaboration the Pastoral Care Department had with the entire hospital's staff, including dining services. In the MICU, chaplains and unit employees worked together to secure "Compassion Carts" for patients and families. Via "Compassion Carts," many ICUs provide family members water, coffee, juice, and nibbles of peanut butter and cheese crackers—or other snacks—while allowing them to remain *in the room* with their loved one. During my residency year, the Compassion Cart became a ritual, always adjacent to the blue-and-white dogwood branch taped to the door—a community symbol of joining the grieving in their impending loss. At hospice, volunteers brought their version of the Compassion Cart to each room—offering sweet treats and hot tea in china cups my Southern mother found charming. One such cart visited us merely an hour before she died.

Sally and I used to talk about the "ritual of touch," as well. During the passing at the hospital of one of her friends, as she and others waited, they all took turns holding his hand and watching the lines on the monitors. At hospice, *reiki* therapists came to Mom's room and offered their energetic touch. I had bawled when one 60-something woman with silver hair and soft eyes had put her hand on my back, and I felt as if she'd released something that had been building in me since the day Mom got sick.

Every hospital and hospice's pastoral care and social work departments, as well as individual units and floors, have a specific protocol and policy for caring for the dying patient and his/her loved ones. From infants, to pediatrics, to adult care, there are resources and support for rituals—from prayer to food to touch to music.

Advance considerations for rituals can be comforting. They may be as simple as prayer, music, family at the bedside, or a "dessert first" policy. As chaplains, Sally and I have come to know those rituals well. And as a family member on the "other side of the curtain," I have learned many new ones—from the routine to the sacred.

Chaplains, of course, are a mainstay of most medium-to-large hospitals, and can be called to visit 24/7. (There is usually an on-call chaplain on site at large hospitals.) Mom also said they were your best resource for care and support, as they could also be a liaison between you and the medical staff. Chaplains know, too, what is available in terms of religious rituals (baptism, blessings, last rites), memorial photos or tangible memory items (such as footprints for infants), as well as spiritual care services (chapel space for prayer, labyrinths for walking, available music/meditation/relaxation, singing bowls, prayer shawls, and Bibles—or other sacred texts [often in Spanish and English]—are available). For those who do not use rituals but seek a way to spiritually care for their dying loved ones, chaplains—as they discern the needs around them—can often provide the basic supports necessary for that situation.

Upon the death of a patient, chaplains can also provide age-specific bereavement materials, as well as local lists of funeral/cremation information (they cannot *recommend* one specific business over another) and support group opportunities for follow-up.

After Mom died, her hospice chaplain arrived at her bedside and offered prayers for her spirit and body. I don't remember what he said, but I remember how comforted I felt in that simple ritual, standing over a lifeless body that, moments early, had held the spirit of my mother. -

From the Practical to the Sacred

From the practical to the personal, Mom taught me and Ron that beginning with the end in mind frees us up, as much as we are able, to *be* with one another at the time of death. Chaplain Sally recalled, during one of our conversations, a recent death of a friend she attended to. Once all the practical health and after-death matters had been handled, she could settle into a rhythm of just *being*.

"After I'd uttered my umpteenth silent prayer for him, I found myself settling into breathing in synch with the machines," she added, and I thought of the beauty of "sharing" the last breaths with those whom we love; even though they are not walking, talking, or really "with us," we touch them, we breathe with them, and we remain close and connected to them for as long as their stay here allows. Touch, presence, and breath are rituals in and of themselves.

The questions we need to ask about care at the end of our lives are essential to determining what we need and want when the time comes—both for our loved ones and ourselves. Talking about them ahead of time allows space for us to embrace whatever time remains—whether death is a seemingly far away possibility, or imminent.

Even when Mom knew the conversation was hard for me and for Ron, she still had it. And it saved many hours of undue terror, stress, and anxiety. We had a plan, and, as soon as she got sick, we put it in gear. It gave us more time to *celebrate* her, to be with her, and to love her.

Because of her forthcoming attitude on death, we also felt invited to keep the conversation light and make jokes. Death need not be gloomy. She always laughed at *Meet the Parents* when Mr. Jinxy peed in the grandmother's ashes; "Don't let Truffy pee on me," she joked. In lieu of pet accidents, Ron and had I opted for a re-enactment of *The Big Lebowski* on Mom's low country "Ashes to Ashes" Road Tour debut. She would have been delighted.

When we prepare ahead of time, and address what we can practically anticipate about death, we potentially have greater opportunity to mine the liminal space between life and death for meaning. Choosing to deal with what we can make preparations for *now*—medical decisions, financial affairs, rituals, readings, music, spiritual items—helps make the actual transition easier from here to whatever's next.

For those of you who *hate* "Freebird," before your family insists on playing it on repeat at your death bed, it would be better for them to know now...rather than when you cannot physically sit up in bed and slap them.

This makes for a much more profound experience of death for everyone—no matter the circumstances. It also helps us savor life. If we consider the end of life to be like its beginning (at birth)—a rite of passage our society and culture considers "worth" spending time planning—then we are invited to offer death—a significant, poignant end to a life well lived—the same, sacred treatment.

Inasmuch as she loved her Scouts Thin Mints and kettle corn, we are invited to take a page out of Mom's book, and always "be prepared."

Chapter 8

Preparing for Death while Savoring Life

"This is what rituals are for. We do spiritual ceremonies as human beings in order to create a safe resting place for our most complicated feelings of joy or trauma."
—Elizabeth Gilbert, Eat, Pray, Love

"On this platform of peace, we can create a language to translate ourselves to ourselves and to each other."
—Maya Angelou, "Amazing Peace: A Christmas Poem"

The Red Notebook

The December before Mom died, she sat on the couch midday in her bathrobe drinking Ghirardelli hot cocoa. This was her usual ritual; she hadn't been dressing or going out much that year. At 77, her physical and mental decline was gnawing at her. Anxiety soared; she bit her lip, scratched her head, and slid her feet back and forth across the carpet profusely—three ticks that always let me know she was stressed.

Having just handed her the hot chocolate, I asked how I might offer her additional help. Maybe, I said, she might want to write in her notebook? (This was one of the ways in which she coped with her manic energy in a body too achy and slow to flitter about.)

"I've been thinking about my memorial service," she added.

"OK, good," I said—trying to hide that I was caught off guard. "Do you want to take a few minutes to write out what you're thinking about?" I suggested.

Energized, she put the hot cocoa down and set pen to paper. She started jotting notes about what she wanted at her memorial service—including hymns, scriptures, time of day. We discussed it briefly over beverages: her, looking worn from dementia and life; me, putting on my best chaplain hat on to hold space and reflect what I heard.

Eight months later, she would die.

How could she have *known* then that her light was dimming?—that she'd lost what one of my professors called "the fire in the belly." Or, as Mom kept saying in those later years, "My get up and go done got up and went." Her writing in the red notebook, with the cup of Ghirardelli beside her, was one of the rituals preparing her, perhaps, for what she already knew was coming.

These are the hardest kinds of rituals, because they require us to think about things that make us uncomfortable. Planning rituals—including determining the details about our own (or loved ones') arrangements, services, and care at the end of life is tough. When we make these conversations special by embracing them intentionally as ritual—a sip of hot cocoa, a discussion over a slow meal, a visit to the space we wish to be buried or scattered—while they're painful, they can also be meaningful.

I will *never* forget that conversation with my mother, both of us sitting on the couch, sipping sweet, dark milk on a bright December midday. As soon as I handed her the notebook, she wrote. As she did so, her anxiety settled. I didn't know it that day, but, with that ritual of hot cocoa and writing, she had invited me into the sacred space of preparing to give her a good death.

Life Is Uncertain; Eat Dessert First

Because neither I nor my mother ever cooked well, people often ask me what I ate growing up. I don't have much recall of our meals, save for "brinner" (breakfast for dinner) and local cafeteria lines.

But what *does* stand out in my memory is my mother's deep love for dessert as ritual. From soothing hot chocolate to cake to pie, to say my mother had a "sweet tooth" is like saying the Dalai Lama *sort of* meditates. Mom was as serious about dessert as "His Holiness" is about his contemplation. For her, the sweetest part of the meal was a *spiritual practice*. This is why she often made it her first or main course, neglecting any nutritional labels we've come to obsess over: carbs, calories, sugars, and saturated fat.

Imploring me to heap *tablespoons* of sugar on my Cheerios and squeeze Hershey's chocolate syrup in my milk, my mother *worshiped* at the altar of refined sugar; she believed in the comforting powers of sweets.

This legacy carried through in all the 36 years I knew her. Whenever Mom, Ron, and I celebrated dinners out for her birthday or other occasions, we knew the drill: restaurants were chosen according to their desserts, not their entrees.

Saint Joseph

Two days before my 37th birthday, I had a dream. It had been seven-and-a-half months since Mom's death. I often prayed that she (or God) would send me messages in my dreams, like the ones I'd had of rummaging through Grandmother Dorothy's drawer. For so many biblical characters I'd read about in Sunday school, dreams seemed important psychologically, spiritually, and theologically; Jacob, Joseph, Pilate's wife—to name a few—had all had meaningful dreams.

By this time, so many rituals were incorporated into my grieving that I began to dream about them. I dreamt that my mother and I were in her car, along with her sister Gail, pulling up to what appeared to be a school or an assisted living facility. Unprompted, Aunt Gail asked Mom what rituals she liked to do on birthdays or anniversaries. Without missing a beat, my mom responded, "I pray to St. Joseph four times with oil."

Well, first, my mother was not Catholic. She had a penchant for sweets, not saints. She was raised Southern Baptist; canonized humans were considered heretical, and anointing was iffy (unless you were one of those mountain Baptists). At this point in the dream, I woke up: 4:45 a.m., alert and refreshed—which is unusual for me. I started the coffee and began to write down the details of the dream, including the symbols that stood out.

The extent of my St. Joseph repertoire is precisely *one instance,* an obscure item: I remembered that one of my best friends, Heather, has another best friend who is Catholic and who buried a statue of St. Joseph in her yard in hopes of selling a house quickly. A little research was needed. I looked up St. Joseph on the Catholic Church's official website, to discover he is the patron saint of workers. But, as I read further, the meaningfulness of his patronage to me and to my mother became apparent: his value as a real estate aid isn't his primary role; he is *first* listed as the patron saint of a happy death. His death is considered happy because the gospels do not refer to him after the beginning of Jesus's public ministry, which suggests he must have died prior.

Throughout the time of the gospels, the early centuries, and until recent history, people generally died at home surrounded by their families (excepting sudden, unexpected, or violent deaths). Tradition has it that because Joseph would have died in the arms of Jesus and Mother Mary, he is therefore perceived as the most blessed human, experiencing a blessed, accompanied death.

St. Joseph's feast day is March 19, one week after my mother's birthday. I kept reading. We are to eat Italian food on his feast day, I discovered, because the Medieval Sicilians prayed to Joseph during a drought and the rains came. On that day, we are to feast to San Giuseppe, Joseph's Italian name—also the name of my parents' favorite restaurant in Clinton, Indiana. Until I read it again on the website that day, the only other place I'd ever read the name "Giuseppe" was on that restaurant sign.

Psychologists will say my brain simply put together these morsels. But in 30-something years, I'd *never* read *anything* about St. Joseph; nor have I ever been curious enough to look him up as "Giuseppe." To say that the shining details—this meta-dream about a ritual—came as an assurance from God would be a stretch for the rational. But to the grieving daughter whose mother died in her arms, a dream that nods to the patron saint of a happy death is mystical, and auspicious, and comforting.

As I considered the dream and its symbolism, I interpreted it as God's giving me my own ritual: a tangible, sacred image or gesture to which we assign meaning. In the dream, when my mother said, "I pray to St. Joseph four times [that day]," I immediately took on her ritual as my own, a faithful assurance that Mom's hospice death had been a peaceful one.

This simple ritual—or a dream about a ritual—gave me a kind of closure after months of anxiety over whether my mother's death had been what she wanted, or whether it had been too painful for her to experience a good death.

And so, through the gifts of that dream, St. Joseph is now the patron saint of this Baptist minister. I invoke him in all my death rituals—including the ways in which I remember Mom, and at the death beds of those I sit and pray with.

When Rituals Matter, and How We Can Do Them

Rituals are the meaning-making stuff of life. They can be tangible—a dessert, an icon or statue of a saint, a holy relic. Or they can transcend the material—as with sacred time, a familiar tune, or an ancient text. They are markers in our journey of life and the path toward, during, and after death, helping us to remember one another in practical and mystical ways.

Rituals are simply about making meaning. Though religious and spiritual traditions may lay claim to them, I don't buy that they are solely religious. Yes, there are certainly rituals and ceremonies within religious or spiritual traditions, but if we try to claim that all rituals *must* reside inside a box of time and place, and under holy authority of a specific entity, we've missed the point.

There are degrees and kinds of rituals, to be sure. Sacraments would qualify as the "high and holy," but they aren't necessarily the rituals I'm focusing on. Rituals for the dying and bereaved do not *require* vestments, ornate liturgy, perfect elocution, traditional accoutrements, or gold-leafed invitations. They can be as simple and understated as a cup of hot cocoa, a pen, and a red notebook—and shouldn't be confused with those other kinds of high church ceremonies.

The ritual may be a one-or-multiple-time occurrence; it may ultimately turn into a tradition. But we need to let go of feeling that a ritual *must* be done formally, properly, in order, without adaptation or spontaneity—all fancy and gilded, long-winded and official—in order to be sacred.

Kate Bowler, navigating her way through the world of cancer diagnosis, treatments, and others' explanations of her suffering, began to understand—to feel—this difference between ritual and care, and ceremony. "I did not tell them how few of their words are needed, but how much their hands are wanted, a hand on my back as I tear up, a hand on my head for a soft prayer of healing. When I feel I'm fading away, these hands prop me up and make me new." Those words continue to remind me what "The Death Squad" members—those chaplains and writers who have journeyed with me on the grief train— continue to teach me: we do not need to be minimizers of pain, the teachers of life lessons, nor the solutions to the problem when it comes to suffering, death, and grief. We need to be the bearers of rituals: creating something sacred in our *presence,* our *silence,* our *touch*—all of which can serve as meaning-making ritual.

The World's Rituals

Formal rituals—from Judaism to Hinduism to Christianity to New Religious Movements—arrive to us in institutional, big-box form. We need look no further than the world's religious and spiritual traditions to see those that are already set in place and ready for use. For many raised in the Christian faith, these are the first kinds of rituals that might be experienced: prayers, baptism, baby dedication, confirmation, and communion.

But when it comes to preparing for death, actively dying, or grieving—traditional, formal rituals may not fit nor fulfill what we need. They also might feel a wee bit confining if we've had any doctrinal or dogmatic challenges within our religious upbringing.

Sometimes, it can feel like religions *own* various rituals, such that we do not feel we have (or we literally do not have) the authority to offer them to ourselves or our loved ones. Certainly, there are many religious rituals that *do* require specific parameters (sacraments, for instance). That said, in life—and in death—there is space for *both:* traditional, formal, religious rituals; and simple, informal, *personal* rituals.

From psalms recited at bedside to ancient prayers, poetry, chanting, healing oils—to candlelit icons of saviors, prophets, and patron saints—we have millennia of humanity's interaction with the Divine to draw upon. (See "Resource 4: Religious, Spiritual, and Sacred Rituals in Preparation for Care at the End of Life and after Death"). These rituals may be for *both* the dying and the bereaved, offering comfort in the mysticism of what Celtic spirituality calls the "thin space" between life and death, as well as for the times the door feels firmly shut, and we (the living) are left behind to grieve.

Rituals for the terminally ill or actively dying can be practiced *any time* within the journey. Rev. Stimp Hawkins held a cardboard-casket-signing party prior to his death. And for nearly a decade prior to his dying he held a gathering each birthday to thank friends and family for another year of support. Long-term or short-term, our rituals help us and our loved ones create sacred space around death. Incorporating rituals infuses what are otherwise heart-wrenching situations with meaning and mysticism. Rituals cannot remove heartbreak, but they can help us cope with it.

The Body as Sacred

Near death, viewing the body's natural "shutting down" processes as sacred rituals in and of themselves can add grace and a level of meaning to dying. I encountered this with Lily as she died in the MICU. As breathing slows (or stops all together) and the color leaves the lips, the warmth and fullness that made that person alive slowly "evaporates." A close observer can see this "evaporation"—it happens very quickly. I liken it to the spirit quietly leaving its temporary home behind. The cessation of breathing and this "evaporation" in and of themselves feel like ritual. The first time I saw someone die—Lily—I experienced this as a mystical aspect of death. I can only describe this as a tiny flutter against my heart, or soul—something deep within me that I've never otherwise had access to except in being present in that moment of death.

Though I've never birthed a child, nor seen one being birthed (in real life), I imagine it's akin to that feeling—for I believe the Universe "shifts" with the beginning or end of a life, and nothing is ever quite the same. In either instance, it feels appropriate to commemorate that moment and acknowledge its meaning. Rituals can do this for us.

Because I didn't know my father was dying until *after* he was already dead, I could not offer King any long-distance *or* bedside rituals. But four days after my father-in-law's cardiac arrest, after he was taken off life support, Fred offered his father a simple Hindu ritual: the quiet recitation of God's name, a chant for the dying. The ritual is intended to keep the loved one's focus on God during death, such that they will receive a new and better birth in which they can continue their spiritual practice and devotion.

Fred's brief, quiet ritual of whispering God's Holy Name in his father's ear before his death, while I stood on the other side of him, is something I count as a ritual given to *both* of our fathers. Though I didn't get to see my father make his transition, in those moments as Great One died, I felt a connection to Daddy. Another lesson I learned from Fred during that time was that, even in the worst circumstances—such as an unexpected death—these rituals demonstrate our faith and help send loved ones off with a mystical, sacred goodbye. (See, again, "Resource 4: Religious, Spiritual, and Sacred Rituals in Preparation for Care at the End of Life and After Death.")

Remembering Our Loved Ones

After bedside rituals for the dying, one of the most powerful things we can continue after our loved ones are no long physically with us is meaning-making *in their absence*. Rituals need not be limited to the bedside. Funerals, memorial services, and times of remembrance are also important rituals to commemorate their lives and legacies. They also aid us in navigating our grief.

At the time when Daddy died suddenly, Fred was only my fiancé, but still accompanied me to Indiana for my father's funeral. Uncle Jon, my father's eldest brother, took care of many of the details. This came as a gift and relief, as I was too shocked to know which way was up. It was only 30 days before the wedding, and my world had suddenly fallen apart. I switched gears quickly—and poorly—from grieving daughter, to bride, and back to grieving daughter again.

My father was born, raised, and died all in Vermillion County. King garnered a particular level of fame through his charisma and stories. My uncle warned us that, prior to the funeral, Daddy's visitation (what some call a wake or viewing) would be an extended event. For *hours* we stood at my father's casket while hundreds of friends trickled through, sharing their memories and favorite stories about Daddy. Despite its length, that ritual of *hearing* others talk about him was so healing for me.

We did not have a visitation nor graveside service for my mother, per her all-caps, underlined request in the red notebook, "NO VISITATION!" and the fact that she was cremated—also her request. But looking back, I wish we still had had that additional ritual, because what I coveted a long time after her death was for people to *talk* about her. During her memorial service, I cried *the entire time.* Start to finish, I sobbed. My uncontrollable blubbering was so severe that I needed to be propped up between Fred and my cousin Britainy, each with their arm around me so that I could remain upright. It was *that bad.*

There was something significant about having a dedicated time for literal "visiting" at my father's visitation that was soothing. The tone of the visitation was less formal; the receiving line allowed us to connect individually with others, hear stories, and cry—or even laugh—and it offered a different kind of support than a more formal time during a funeral would. While we honored my mother's request for no visitation, I learned that *grief* rituals are for those who have to carry on without the physical presence of their loved ones, so it's important—while being respectful—to do what *we need to do* for our healing.

"Funerals are for the living," my mother said once, decades ago.

During the reception portion after her memorial service, many folks shared their memories about my mom. It wasn't the same, though. After the service, I was exhausted. At the reception portion, gracious church folk were concerned about checking on my well-being, rather than telling stories or sharing memories of Mom. I learned that even though you're tired and grieving, it's important to hold as much space as possible for others to show their support, love, and compassion through the ritual of community gathering and remembrances—whether through visitations, wakes, viewings, funerals, memorials, graveside services, or receptions. Dedicating a time to remembrance, meaning-making, and lifting up one's beloveds up is nothing less than soul-stirring, important work.

Many times, I've witnessed families rush to complete the services (often due to travel, circumstances, and the practical logistics of finances and the perishable nature of our bodies). Or they skip them all together. But we *need* our time and space to grieve publicly—and it doesn't need to be complex. It's not a wedding; no fancy service, nor printed programs are required for gathering together to *remember.* When our loved ones die, we're exhausted, sad, fearful, stoic. There are a million reasons we think it will be easier to take care of things quickly, briefly, and cheaply. But I recommend this: relish any and all time in public remembrance; seize opportunities for visitations, wakes, receiving lines, memorial services, funerals, graveside services. Those help us begin and continue our grief process; they give us rituals whose meanings we may not understand in the planning, but fully appreciate when they are enacted.

Bury Me at Honey Creek Square

"Bury me at Honey Creek Square," my father would sing to me at an early age, making fun of consumerists obsessed with the only shopping mall within a 30-minute radius of our tiny western Indiana county. King had no interest in fancy stores. He didn't amuse himself to death with retail therapy, and he caricatured those who did. He was *at home* in the corn fields.

And so, we buried him in Bono Cemetery, a few miles outside of his hometown of Dana, Indiana. He was laid to rest beside my paternal grandparents, in a peaceful plot they had purchased for him decades ago—when they must have anticipated he'd die alone. The three of them rest there now, with 360° views of the lush green corn rows whose fall harvest leaves them looking like dark corduroy pants. I imagine my father and grandparents loving taking in the Midwest's unconstructed sunrises and sunsets.

A local military color guard was present at my father's graveside. They offered a 21-gun salute and handed me a folded flag. It was a simple, formal ritual—but profound.

My father's devotees, of which he had many, attended the viewing, funeral, and military graveside burial. They were just as loyal in his death as they had been during his life. Though they didn't understand all the complexities of our relationship, they knew they didn't need to. They understood my place as his daughter, and so they were fiercely loyal to me, too. Goathead, one of my father's best friends, promised to inflict serious bodily injury on Fred if he ever hurt me. Fred took him at his word; Daddy's weathered friends look too coarse not to be taken at their word.

A year later, I was a co-officiant for Fred's father's memorial service. His pastor and I invited attendees to offer stories about his work and friends, about his affinity for milk (he drank at least two gallons per week) and his relentless teasing of me for my conversion to vegetarianism. Co-workers spoke of his problem-solving skills, including the time he got a broken-down vehicle back on the road by putting a sock in the carburetor. We reminded everyone what they already knew: "Great One" was a hard-working provider for his family, and a good, Christian man. All of these are the kinds of stories we *need* to hear in grief, so we know that our loved ones *will be remembered* for their character and their quirks.

Holy Memories, Holy Relics

Grief rituals come in all shapes and sizes—from the traditional to the seemingly strange, or even the mundane. When Fred completes some engineering feat, I remind him that "Great One" would be very proud. When I'm telling a dramatic story and over-emphasizing details for effect, Fred reminds me that I am my father's daughter.

When I complain about something completely irrational and often a First World problem, Fred does his best impression of my mother, whose "princess" tendencies often left her unsatisfied in even the most ideal situations.

Instantly, our parents are seated at the dinner table with us; it's an informal ritual of remembering them as real people—not saints nor sinners, but the actual loved ones we will always miss.

Years before she died, my paternal grandmother wrote a long, handwritten note and stuffed it into her underwear drawer, where we discovered it after her death. By her writing those words, she also created a ritual repeated for years to come, in which each of her descendants would sit at the kitchen table, silently staring at a blue-felt–backed, plastic tablecloth she always used, hearing her voice as those inked words were read aloud from the notebook paper.

This was the ritual she created: she wanted her people to gather at her table while she told us all the things we needed to hear—including all the "holy relics" precious to her that she wanted each of us, by name, to have/use/wear to remember her by. On that day long ago, when death was a mere distant acquaintance, she fashioned a ritual that would become one of the most meaningful family rituals we have.

Similarly, my mother's best friend (and my second mother), Mama Phyllis created another ritual. One afternoon, when I drove to Burlington to visit her and she was still well enough to move about the house, she said, "Come on," and waved me on to follow her from the kitchen breakfast nook into each room of the house.

"You tell me exactly what you want," she said, as we entered each room. I froze. *What was I supposed to say?* She knew it had taken me by surprise, so she made suggestions; at the end of the "tour," we sat on the couch and made the list. Several years later, three young men and I loaded up the "The Healing Room" and drove it to Raleigh. The Healing Room was the front guest bedroom in Phyllis's brick ranch home. The Healing Room contained her grandparents' bedroom suite, probably purchased just after the turn of the last century. My mother gave this room its name, because we'd drive the 30 minutes from the town we lived in to stay with Phyllis for a few days, and those were always days of healing for us. That room was always open, ready to accept worn-out pilgrims in need of rest and recovery.

Several lifetimes of memories were contained in this one room, now loaded onto a truck, to be added to a grieving 32-year-old's apartment. How do our lives end up like this? Relics we've cherished, divided among those whom we cherished, in hopes that our smells and faces will last far beyond the erasure of time.

When the furniture arrived, everything from the "Healing Room" smelled like Phyllis—from her green butterfly purse to her parents' chest of drawers. Every time I see the three brass candlesticks from her that I stationed on my mantel, I'm instantly transported to her living room, where I spent so much of my childhood, and passed the last afternoons of her cancer journey talking to her about anything but dying: her, lying on the loveseat asking for stories about *real life*,…and me, trying not to imagine the day when she wouldn't be around to ask for more stories.

And yet we all end up here: burying our loved ones, gripped by the things they leave behind, praying their spirits will remain close, and that their Chanel No. 5 will cling to us. Their voices haunt us; their smiles linger in our minds—like the one from that sunny afternoon when I took a mental snapshot of her, tired but happy for my company.

The joke is always on us, because we love, love, love, and yet everyone we try so desperately to hold on to dies, dies, dies.

But we keep these holy relics in our own living rooms, making rituals out of blowing kisses to photographs, wearing their jewelry, and thinking to ourselves, "My God, I hope *someone* misses me this much when I'm gone."

The Healing Room is now with me, in hopes that it will heal my loss. Even after death, Phyllis still gives her comfort.

Chapter 9

Putting the Fun in FUNeral

*"And what is it to cease breathing, but to free the breath
from its restless tides, that it may rise and expand
and seek God unencumbered?"*
—Khalil Gibran, "On Death," The Prophet

Let's Talk about Boobs

The word Americans fear most is not *terrorist*, nor is it *murderer*. The word that brings people to their knees quicker than a hostage standoff is *cancer*. The "C" word is a ubiquitous, silent, and horrifying killer, because it's sneaky, like that big hairy spider you swore was there just a minute ago when you left to get that paper towel to (gently) squeeze him to his timely death. *Where is it now?* you think. *Oh, dear Lord Jesus.*

Every six months for nearly two years, I've been getting mammograms. It's a little early for a woman my age, but appropriate given new symptoms starting about two years ago in what I affectionately call my "troublesome boob."

I'm grateful for modern medical diagnostic equipment, with its fancy robotic X-ray arms and 3-D capabilities. That's awe-inspiring. But the part that's the weirdest, and *scariest*, thing about a mammogram is the *waiting room*.

The mammogram waiting room is 800 square feet of trembling anxiety. We ladies sit in our fuchsia muumuus—braless, and one wardrobe malfunction away from a nip-slip—and, yet, we stare at our phones, pretending as if fancy pedicures await us. Then, after we've completed our routine mammogram, we return to the *waiting room*, to await a radiology tech, who comes up and whispers one of two phrases:

"You're free to go, sweetheart! See you next year!"...*or*...

"The radiologist would like to take a few more pictures, dear. Follow me."

Everyone wants the former.

I always get the latter.

When you spend three hours in the Pepto Bismol Bull Pen, you worry *a lot*. You hear *a lot*. Women come and go to the soundtrack of ultrasound room chatter from down the hall and endless rounds of "Hold your breath!" To be fair, they provide free coffee and tea, but when we're already juggling a purse and a plastic hospital bag full of our "belongings," there's an urgency to pack light. No one wants a Styrofoam cup of boiling beverage to keep them from running for the dressing room as soon as clearance arrives.

I've seen women leave the office with glee. Others slump out, twilight-zoned because they've heard the "C" word, or, "We need further tests" (often code for biopsy). One never leaves the mammography suite knowing exactly what has happened unless Trish the Tech whispers in her angelic tone, "Free to go, hon!"

I've heard the "C" word, the "B" word, and everything in between. And yet, "nothing definitive." I don't have cancer, but for 24 months I've had the "troublesome boob." It reminds me that we all live with some form of the "D Word," the "C" word, even if at certain points we're "free to go, hon," we *never* really know what could happen next.

The Death Rate Is 100 Percent

As someone who teaches college students in their late teens or early 20s, I've been given the opportunity to interact with a group of people who, for the most part, imagine themselves to be invincible and indestructible, much like I felt at their age. There is no recreational drug that will conquer them, no amount of alcohol that can claim their lives, no texting-while-driving that will smash their bodies against crumpled steel. And they don't like to engage in any future-scenario thinking in which they do not live forever.

Part of my job is to gently remind them: "You're going to die."

They guffaw at such absurdity. I add: "I'm going to die, too."

"What?!" they respond. "Quit playing. Don't say that." They are dear and loving, and don't want to walk in one day to discover the one who cheerleads them through to finals is no longer there.

"It's true; better start thinking about it now."

They peg me as dramatic.

But in our World Religions course, during which we ponder all the spiritual traditions and their "Ultimate Purpose," they begin to finally imagine the possibility—because they see that our ancestors tried to figure it out, too. Week after week, we read texts on theology, faith, rituals, and the ways in which ancient and modern peoples have considered what comes next.

As they allow themselves to learn and be shaped and formed by these global traditions, they begin to understand how humanity—across time and place—has prepared and planned for the great beyond.

Putting the Fun in FUNeral

For over 14 years I've been an unwitting student of death, seeing hundreds of deaths and losing nine close loved ones— including my father, my mother, my father-in-law, and aunts and uncles and grandparents. But for many of these years, I hadn't (yet) given much thought to my *own* death.

Then, one day, while driving I-40 eastbound in the right lane at 65 mph, a thought came over me, with no warning:

You could die, Dana. Like, right now. *You know that, right?*

My mother hadn't died yet; I wasn't actively grieving a loved one. I wasn't even consciously thinking of death. I was listening to "Cheerleader," an upbeat, moderate-tempo song with an ear-worm chorus.

If you died right now—on I-40, it would be OK. You know why? You've had a wonderful life, Dana. You really have.

I really had, up to that point. And I *still* really have, up to this one.

I *didn't* die that night on the highway (obviously), but, like an omen, it signaled that my world was shifting, and I needed to think on these things. Then, months later, Mom got sick and died. Death inched closer and closer.

One night, over tacos, I decided it was time to give Fred my plan.

After his father died, Fred briefly told me his death plan. It's simple and reflects his monastic roots: a peaceful death with pain management. He wants to be enveloped by hearing his favorite scripture and *kirtan* (call-and-response devotional singing). We are all to chant the "Holy Name" he chanted for his father.

In between bites of our taco dinner, as I wiped salsa from my face, I sketched my own plan out for him, and it was more... complex—something more similar to a concert rider for a diva.

To begin, if I'm served a terminal diagnosis with a side of timelines, call the palliative care doctors first; inpatient or outpatient hospice is next. Pain meds are to be distributed *generously*. And I don't want to be left alone at night. (Because of the nature of such demands on my loved ones, I encouraged Fred to keep my death vigil short and sweet, so he wouldn't have to camp out too long.)

"Please make me smell good," I told him, saying this is of utmost importance, while explaining the mixture of lavender oil I want sprayed on me, around me, and on anything standing still.

"Brush my teeth, put on a little deodorant, and rub me with peppermint lotion," I directed. "I want to smell good, so folks will get close, touch me, hug me, and kiss me."

"Touches," he responded, pretending to make a mental note.

"*Anybody* can come visit," I added. I've had so many patients and family members say, "I don't want anyone to see me like *that*." That is not the case for me. I *love* people, and even if I only have two friends left to my name by that time, I want them both buzzing around me in those final days. But I also respect that it may be painful for some people to see a dying person. "In that case," I told Fred, "tell them to feel free to call; place the phone to my ear and I'll listen all day."

"And I want lots of prayer: Taizé and scripture; add some fancy reiki for you, or whatever else you need," I added, realizing, after my inpatient hospice experience with Mom, some of the care instructions should be designed to attend to the exhausted caregivers.

"But no dogs! Lord Jesus, no dogs!" I added, remembering a Buddhist nun telling me that any animal present at the time of death influences the body (human or animal) the departed will take in the next life.

"What about cats?" He asked.

"*Purrrrfect*," I instructed, because if reincarnation is the way God has worked this all out, a cat's life would be my dream.

"Stay with me as I die if you can," I continued to boss him.

"Do you want to die at home, or the hospital, or hospice?" he asked, beginning to take notes at this point.

"Hospital or hospice—no home," I told him, only because I *know* the trauma of dying at home, and how it hard it is to visit or live there again. Nothing ever looks or feels the same way.

"Please also make certain I'm dead... I mean, like, *really* dead before they roll me away," I instructed.

"Sternal rub?" He grinned, remembering Ron's trick with Mom.

He made a fist with his right hand and rubbed his knuckles against my sternum (because he knows it drives me crazy—at least while I'm alive).

"Ow! *STOP!*" I pushed his hand away.

"Please cremate me with some cool, holy relics you don't mind parting with" I added, remembering how rosy and peaceful Mom had looked with her prayer shawl tucked under her chin, hands folded neatly on her belly, with the Christian prayer beads and a Hindu tulsi necklace wrapped around her wrist.

"Feel free to ask for any gold teeth," I offered, "before they put me in."

"In?" Fred asked.

"In the cremation oven."

"You're so irreverent," Fred said.

"No! Seriously—melt them down, cash them out, and donate the money to charity; let it make a difference.

"But I *would* like a party," I added. "A good one—like with kettle corn, garlic knots, sweet tea, and Kombucha for the hipsters," I explained, naming my favorite foods.

"I'll write my obituary and the liturgy for you ahead of time," I told him, and he began to realize I *was* planning my own funeral (or FUN-eral, as I've begun calling it since I first came upon the term). For, though I'm only in my late 30s, have no terminal illness (though I do have a "troublesome boob"), and no impending "sense of doom" that I am going to die next week, I still don't want him burdened with pulling things together. Plus,...I'm bossy.

I want to be cremated, even though many Christians question this decision due to confusing scriptures on bodily resurrection. I do not wish to take up valuable land/space in a cemetery no one will visit. Yes, I'm claustrophobic. Yes, I'm terrified of fire. But I'm impatient too; I'd much rather get it over with quickly than hang out in the ground for years as a worm buffet *waiting* to become dust. Plus, I'd like to be scattered at the three "Bs": Binkley, Bono, and "the Beach," with a little saved if Fred (or anyone else) wants me buckled in their passenger seat or guarding the living room from intruders.

"Use Mama Phyllis's ginger jar from the fireplace mantel, and recess me from the sanctuary to the Fellowship Hall while playing 'Back in Black,'" and Fred laughed, realizing I was being both silly and serious.

"You know, then, to scatter me at the three Bs," I reminded him. "Recite them for me," I said, as he rolled his eyes. "Just humor me," I implored.

But he has become well-versed in this particular part, as we discussed where we wanted our ashes placed when we completed our estate paperwork.

"Binkley, Beach, and Bono?"

"Yep," I confirmed. Binkley is our church; a beach is any of his choosing, and Bono is the western Indiana corn field where my father and grandparents are buried. Ideally, I'd like a road trip retracing the stops of Mom's Ashes-to-Ashes Tour, but I realize that's a lot to ask.

Fred and I have since gone through each item he's planned (or at least started to plan) or needed, should my death be next week. Legal papers have long been signed. (A brief overview of such similar basic paperwork can be found in: "Resource 2: Practical and Legal Preparations").

I have an obituary saved on my computer. It's verbose and grandiose, yes, but it makes it easy for Fred to cut-and-paste onto whatever clunky memorial website the crematorium sets up for him. (See "Resource 5: Practical Considerations *after* Death.")

From obituary to services, ash-scattering to legacy, I've left him with a sketch, so that, in his grief, he doesn't have to start with a blank page. At this point in our marriage, our conversations about death remain light. Neither one of us has a diagnosis—though we remember, as Kate Bowler stated, "We're all terminal." Most days I tell Fred that I still see death as a distant destination, and thus I can approach it with some levity. But the irony is: each day I say it, the destination comes closer.

At 37, I've been loved, educated, and done the two things I *always dreamt of doing:* writing and teaching. I was born to two of the (literally) craziest parents ever, who loved me despite their mental illnesses and penchant for intoxicating substances. I was raised by grandparents and aunts and uncles who cheered me before I knew how badly I needed it. I have a brother and sister-in-law who have empowered me to be independent, capable, and to embrace my gifts. I've lived to see my niece and nephew be born, grow up, and become successful. My two paternal first cousins have been just like my own sisters, and I have many more best friends than I've ever deserved. I married my soul mate and we travel well together. I've *felt* love, and, more importantly, have been blessed to *give* love.

I've met and taught students from many states, nations, and circumstances. I've worshiped in all flavors of Christian churches, Jewish synagogues, Hindu temples, mosques, and Buddhist centers. It's been a wonderful life, indeed.

On my best days, I embrace this wholeheartedly; on my worst days, I'm scared *to death* of death—hanging on for dear life, clawing and clinging to people and things and begging God to let me see the year 2,100. (I'd be 119.).

At the end of most days, I feel gratitude for the very full life I've lived—nearly 11 years of which have been spent knowing Fred. "Should I die before I finish this book," I tell him (or before my 40th, or 50th, birthday), "it's OK," I add, "Because God has given me the most circuitous, holy, wild ride ever. I wouldn't change a thing."

Writing this book has been reinforcing of this realization: my hospital chaplaincy, our fathers' deaths, and all the loss I've experienced taught me how to give Mom "a good death." This compounding of lessons all led up to coping with the most important death: Mom's. The book has come from laughing *and* crying *and* grieving. It came from living without our beloved ones who've seemingly vanished behind a curtain that some days feels thick and heavy—like they never even existed. Other days, the veil is light and thin—like they've never left.

Epilogue

Ashes to Ashes Road Tour

My grief journey was at the forefront of the first year without Mom. Her ashes have rested on our mantel, in our bedroom, in the kitchen, near my laptop, and in my car. And with Undertaker Jake's seatbelt inspiration, Mom has traveled extensively.

Since we began her road tour on the beach during a gale-force wind warning on what would have been her 78th birthday, I haven't hesitated to buckle her in. Tiny traces of Mom have been scattered here and there, including undisclosed public parks (*sorry!*) and on loved ones' tombstones. Wherever the road took us, I took a photo. From sand to granite, I commemorated her Sunset Scatter Box wherever its "issuance" was spread.

"She's surprisingly photogenic," Fred once said of her ashes, when I showed him photos of Mom's box in her hometown on her parents' and siblings' graves. That destination made me a little nervous; their cemetery is located just off a busy road, where I could easily have been discovered.

What in the name of all that is holy is that crazy woman doing? I imagined a passerby saying just before they called the cops.

That's the same cemetery where Mom taught me to drive (not a good idea). While in reverse, I knocked over someone's granite memorial bench. I was 14; we were broke. So, I got a special permit to work for minimum wage as a Winn-Dixie grocery bagger to earn the money pay for the damage. Once I paid it off, Mom insisted on *taking my photo* while posing on bench.

"It's yours now," she laughed. "You earned it."

She gave a copy of the photo to my driver's ed teacher.

Though I don't have the *best* reputation in that hometown cemetery, I still scattered and snapped photos. Don't tell anyone.

Countless people have likely seen me parked or driving around with a box of cremated ashes strapped into my passenger seat. There's no telling what runs through their heads when they see "Mom" while at the gas pump or in the grocery store parking lot. I do know this: *no one* is going to steal a Civic with a dead person riding shotgun.

I haven't yet mustered up the courage to take her through the Wendy's drive-thru for a Frosty, but I know she's waiting for it.

"Dessert *first*," she'd insist.

Practical and Spiritual Resources

Introduction: How to Use These Resources

We are all terminal. This is not a curse; rather, knowing that we are finite and mortal offers us an invitation for preparation and making-meaning. My aim for your reading of this book and learning more about death, dying, and grief, is to support you in taking action on three things:

- *first,* understanding your own mortality and planning for your end-of-life care;

- *second,* sharing your plan with someone who can advocate your wishes for you;

- *third,* helping someone else do the same.

Starting this conversation with ourselves and others is tough. When something is awkward or disappointing, feel free to pat yourself on the back for bravely speaking up—and, feel free to add in a little humor when it doesn't work according to plan. (As my father used to say, "Well, that went over like a turd in a punch bowl.")

Please know that I *know* this is hard.

Facing these truths—and doing something—is never easy. When we embrace the fact that we—and our loved ones—die, we truly have the freedom to *live*. When we prepare for death while savoring life, we begin with the end in mind. Life, then, becomes precious and sweet—just like *dessert first!*—not merely something we're muddling through.

The following resources help us navigate explorations and conversations about death, dying, and grief. They broadly fit into the following categories: conversation starters, practical and legal preparations, religious and spiritual preparations, grieving, theological wonderings, and additional scriptural, book, and endnotes resources. The legal aspects are those questions that must be answered in accordance with each state's laws and the medical care we want (or do not want) to receive when the time comes. (Note that I did not type "if"; try to embrace "when.")

Depending upon your unique circumstances, the legal and/ or medical preparations might be the most pressing for you and your loved ones. From estate distribution wishes to medical forms, having our "papers" or "affairs" in order is of utmost importance, particularly if we want to ensure that we—and our loved ones— have our wishes honored.

It was in this spirit that Rev. "Stimp" Hawkins—"The Death Pimp"—carried his "papers" *with* him 24/7. You needn't do that—but, at the very least, a simple conversation is useful for helping your loved ones *know* what you'd like for them to do in an emergency. *Legal* medical forms guide emergency personnel as to our wishes, should our loved ones *not* be present to convey them for us.

Now, if we are healthy and 8, 18, or 48, it is *certainly* appropriate that *everything* that can be done medically should be done to intervene to save us. But if we are 78 or 108, with a terminal diagnosis, we may *not want* extreme, curative medical interventions for our bodies. Therefore, we (and our loved ones) must explore the possibilities and have "the conversation"— about practical medical matters—and beyond.

We don't have to get all this right or perfect; we simply need to get *started*. Whether it's considering legal paperwork, emergency decisions, end-of-life planning, or grieving, here are some basic steps to help us *begin*. Now's the time for us to all channel our inner Frank Sinatra: "I did it *myyyy* way."

Resource 1

Conversation Starters

Working on acknowledging and honoring our own losses—our grief trains—can be a good first step in preparing for any impending loss. This includes how we help prepare our loved ones—practically and spiritually—to care for us at the end of life, and grieve us well. But talking about illness, death, and loss feels "icky." We are often quick to shut down the topic, minimize it, and move along quickly. But remember, we would *never* minimize an infant's birth or a child's adoption. We spend months planning for these new lives. Why not invest a little time on the *end* of life—which is as certain as its beginning?

Here are some conversation starters with loved ones:

Strategy #1: Blame it on this author. "So, I've been reading this book and this crazy lady actually *plans* her own funeral and the kind of care she wants when she's dying. She's *only* 37 when she does this. Crazy, huh? It's weird, but, it made me think about..."

Strategy #2: Blame it on friends or lawyers. "Well, Donna and I and had dinner with Tammy and Jeff last week. They had just been to visit a lawyer to get their affairs in order. S/he said that we should get our paperwork together for *our* wills, and decide who should hold our health-care power of attorney. Apparently, it's a mess if you don't have all that outlined in advance, so I've been thinking about it—and I want to share some things with you..."

Strategy #3: Recall a recent death of a loved one, and how they did have their paperwork and care planned out—or didn't—and how others around them felt/coped. "You know, when Grandmother died, it was so helpful that she had told us what she wanted at her funeral. I'm glad she did that, so that we could give her the best send-off possible. I'd like to do that for myself and for you. May we talk about **that for a few minutes, please?**"

Strategy #4: Be honest. "I'd like to take some time to share my wishes with you about care for the end of my life. Now, I don't plan on dying any time soon, but I want you to know what I want so that you don't have to make any tough decisions—you'll know exactly what I want, and all you'll have to do is advocate if I can't for myself. And I want to be able to do the same for you. **OR,** "Mom/Dad/Grandma/Grandpa, I know it's hard to think about the end of our lives, but I want you to know that I am here for you, and I want to make informed decisions about what *you* want should you have an emergency. May we please talk about that for a few minutes so I'll know how to take care of you if the need arises?"

Resource 2

Practical and Legal Preparations

This list is not necessarily exhaustive. Not *everything* needs to be tackled all at once. If death is *not* imminent (by this, I mean within the next week or month), *take your time and attend to these in bite-sized segments*. Five or ten minutes at a time is *plenty*. Keep a notebook or folder with the list where you can sketch out details, or keep this book where you can reach it easily to jot down notes as they occur or result from conversations, events, or appointments with loved ones.

A lawyer and your primary care physician can both be *very* helpful in securing and completing paperwork. Fred and I completed age-appropriate legal forms in our early 30s. Our local credit union offered estate attorney services at a reduced rate. The entire process took only several hours. Each state has different laws regarding legally binding paperwork. Be sure to check government websites for suggested forms. There is also an age requirement for completing these forms, which is usually 18 or over.

Suggested Legal and Medical Paperwork to Secure and Complete

Completing the basic legal paperwork for care and financial decisions is the highest priority. Such paperwork includes power of attorney and health-care power of attorney forms, advance directives (living will), will and estate documents. These are what you and your loved ones will need to have in place in order to make medical care and financial decisions.

Basic Care Paperwork: The following are specific to medical care and must be discussed with a physician if and when age/medically appropriate.

— DNR: Do Not Resuscitate order—this means that you are to receive no CPR in the event of a cardiac and/or respiratory arrest.

— DNI: Do Not Intubate order—this means that you are not to receive a breathing tube in the event of a respiratory arrest.

— M.O.S.T. Form: "Medical Orders for Scope of Treatment"— this is a much more detailed outline of wishes for treatment in a medical emergency or event. It includes options such as oxygen, medications, feeding tubes, etc.

Connect with Local Medical Resources

• *Palliative Care* simply means comfort care. This involves wishes regarding pain and comfort management at the end of life, when all curative (life-saving) treatment has ceased. While this typically does not require a specific form, you may wish to contact your local hospice organization for suggestions on what can be planned in advance. (See "Hospice" immediately following.) In addition, *write down your wishes*, or express them to whoever will oversee your care at the end of life. Whomever you choose to have your health-care power of attorney should be informed of these wishes.

• *Hospice:* Feel free to connect with your county or city's local hospice organization regarding services and requirements for inpatient and outpatient (at-home) care. Both palliative and hospice care options may be discussed with your primary physician if age/medically appropriate.

• *Organ Donation:* Most local DMVs provide the opportunity to add an organ donor heart to your license or identification card at your request. I've added the heart on mine and discussed with Fred and Ron, who has my health-care power of attorney, that I would, indeed, like my organs donated if they can be used. You may also wish to contact a local organ donation service to discuss any additional details regarding the process.

Additional Suggested Practical Considerations for Preparation

• *Passwords, Passcodes, and Banking:* This is a more pressing issue today than even just a decade ago. The ability to log into smartphones, email, banking accounts—or to secure medical information quickly (e.g., prescriptions, allergies, medical history)—can be essential if we or a loved one becomes ill or dies suddenly. Having access to passwords, passcodes, and/or keys to safety deposit boxes or safes that contain paperwork is essential. We must be certain that our family, spouse, partner, best friends, person granted our power of attorney (and/or health-care power of attorney), or whomever we wish to handle our affairs in an emergency or in the case of death has access to these.

- *Partner/Spouse:* Do keep in mind that while you may wish your partner or spouse to be your designated go-to person in a medical crisis, there may be a situation in which they are unable to do so. (Imagine if they were in a serious car accident *with* you.) In this case, keep in mind an additional person (sibling, family member, best friend) whom you would like to act on your behalf should your partner/spouse be unable to. Also, keep this in mind for your partner/spouse, should you be incapacitated and unable to advocate for *them.*

General Preparation for Care at the End of Life

The following are less formal considerations, but equally as important. They may be shared over hot cocoa with a loved one, jotted down in a notebook, or merely mentioned over the phone. The point of the following questions is for us—and our loved ones—to begin with the end in mind. Thinking through some of these preferences *now* helps us and our loved ones prepare to offer us a "good death"—one in which we can savor the remaining moments of life.

- Ideally, where would you like to die?

- Whom would you like to be there / have visit? (e.g., loved ones or pets)

- What atmosphere is preferable? (e.g, quiet, busy with visitors, or other)

- How would you prefer to rest during your transition? (e.g., in a medical bed, in your own bed, or in a favorite chair or sofa)

- What sounds would be pleasing to you? (e.g., favorite music, sacred music, favorite instrument, loved ones' voices, loved ones' story-telling, laughter, prayer, singing bowls, nature sounds, white noise, silence)

- What smells would be pleasing to you, if any (e.g., parfum, candles, scents of favorite foods, essential oils)

- What sights would be pleasing to you (e.g., artificial lighting, sunlight, nature, photos of loved ones and/or pets, movies, favorite art, travel photography, etc.)

- What touch (if any) would be pleasing to you (e.g., hugs, hand-holding, gentle back rub or massage, or no touch)?

- What kind of care do you prefer for your body? (e.g., lotion, massage oil, ritual cleansing, hygiene preferences [bathing, dental], cosmetic practices such as make-up, clothing)

Resource 4

Religious, Spiritual, and Sacred Rituals in Preparation for Care at the End of Life and after Death

Rituals—whether formal, informal, religious, or spiritual—help add meaning-making moments to life's (and death's) most important times. As with the rituals covered in previous chapters, they needn't be fancy or by-the-book. They can be active *or* passive—things we *do* or things that *engage* our senses. Here are some questions to help you consider what may help you (and others) make meaning at the end of life:

- What religion and/or spiritual sights would be pleasing to you? (e.g., religious iconography, pictures of a religious figure [Christ, a particular saint, guru, teacher, the Pope])

- What religious and/or spiritual sounds would be pleasing to you? (e.g., favorite recordings, gospel music, hymn singing, chanting, mantra meditation)

- What religious rituals would you like to occur, if any, during your end-of-life transition? (e.g., Catholic sacrament of Last Rites; reading from a specific sacred liturgy, text, or prayer book; sitting *shiva*; singing; poetry reading; scripture reading; kirtan; mantra chanting; extemporaneous prayers; or other)

- Are there other rituals within your religious, spiritual, cultural, ethnic, or family traditions to be considered *immediately following death?* (e.g., ritual washing, prayers recited, a particular "send-off")

Practical Considerations after Death

These are practical—from the typical to the unusual—considerations for the body immediately following death. Yes, it may seem morbid to think about *the dead body*, but these are very real questions.

Do you want an autopsy and/or to donate your entire body?

- Because she was a nurse, mom *swooned* at the idea of being a medical school cadaver. She had, and Ron has, a stomach of steel; they could both easily talk autopsies over oatmeal. Had we had more logistical time, we *may* have been able to arrange for this donation, but I'm not certain, since we didn't investigate it fully. I do wish, though, that we'd spent a bit more time talking about it with her, so that we could have actually determined if her wish could have been fulfilled, rather than her merely joking about her body being a useful "teacher" for a future medical professional.

- Fred's father *did* have an autopsy prior to his cremation. Because he was found unconscious in unusual circumstances (a family reunion), and perhaps because we (his family) looked rather suspicious, Great One was a "Medical Examiner Case." This meant that the ME (Medical Examiner) had jurisdiction over his body until the cause of death could be determined. This *could* have felt disturbing; however, it wasn't, because we were all anxious to know what, precisely, had happened to him. Fred and his brother felt it necessary and useful for death certificate information and beyond, and as costs for ME cases such as this are covered by the hospital, there was no additional charge to the family.

- Families often opt out of an autopsy if there isn't more *urgent* information to glean about a loved one's condition. For my brother and for me, we knew there would likely be an additional cost and, perhaps, a wait. So now I tell people that, *if* an autopsy is important to them, they should advocate for this upfront. I now wish we had honored Mom's wish to be "donated to science," and I also wish I'd advocated for an autopsy for my own father, as his cardiac arrest was "complex."

What funeral home service or crematorium would you like to be used?

Would you like a burial or cremation? Is there anything in particular that you'd like to be buried or cremated in/with? For instance, do you have a preferred outfit for your funeral (burial), or a holy relic you'd like to be cremated with? Mom was cremated with a prayer shawl knitted by a friend, glass prayer beads from the Christian tradition, and wooden prayer beads from the Hindu tradition.

Would you like to be embalmed or not? Note: Cremated individuals can also choose to be embalmed prior to cremation.

If burial, would you like an open casket service, or not?

(If applicable) Would you like a masonic funeral, military funeral, and/ or 21-gun salute?

Services Preference: Visitation, wake, reception, funeral, memorial, graveside service, columbarium service, ashes scattering, interment of ashes, or other?

Services Logistics: Where would you like your services to be held? I've seen everything—from houses of worship to hospital chapels to cemeteries to favorite restaurants to beaches to nonprofit organizations to college campuses. Anything goes, so long as the location is available. The biggest considerations are: where it is to take place, and whom you would like invited.

— Whom would you like to officiate or speak at your service, if anyone? (e.g., clergy, family/friends sharing)

— Do you have in mind any specifics aspects for your service? (e.g., religious readings, poetic readings, special music, etc.)

— Is there anything you'd prefer your loved ones *not* do at your service?

What would you like for your loved ones to do following your service? (e.g., reception, dinner, party, receive friends and guests at the home)

Formal and Legal Considerations

Obituary

Printed newspaper obituaries have become criminally expensive. A small, short obituary with just the facts can run a family upwards of $600. Most funeral homes and crematoriums factor a full obituary into their packages, but keep in mind they usually place a short death notice in the local paper as part of their services, too. As newspapers near extinction, memorial pages have replaced the paper obituary. What I love most about these sites is that they come ready-made, usually through the funeral home or crematory services, and are easy to prepare and edit.

A longer obituary can be written and placed on the website, where viewers can leave memories and notes for the bereaved. The website lives on in perpetuity, providing a source of comfort (and family history).

There are many ways to write an obituary, including short and sweet or clever and funny. Unless you are a professional obit writer for *The New York Times,* there are no rules, but I suggest focusing on respect and honesty. If you make stuff up, it can be confusing to the historical records and for family members reading it decades later. Obituaries can be narrative, or just the facts. This can be left up to you and your family to determine how you'd like to write it if you determine to do it on your own. For an additional (sometimes prohibitive) cost, funeral homes offer different packages that may include writing an obituary for you.

Death Certificates and Estate Processes

There are many legal considerations following a loved one's death. This can all be *very* overwhelming mid-grief, so pre-planning is most useful. Funeral homes and crematoriums will assist in completing the *immediate* required legal information for a death certificate. Be certain to order several *original* copies (a minimum of five), as many organizations require an original death certificate for financial accounts, estate processes, retirement funds, social security, and life insurance.

Resource 6

Stimp (The Death Pimp) and Martha's Lessons on Savoring Life while Preparing for Death and after Death

Lesson 1. *Start the Conversation*

Stimp was amazing to me, because of his interest in beginning with the end in mind. Were he still physically with us, I'm sure he'd be the first to read and share this book. He'd probably even suggest a "Death Chaplain and Death Pimp" road tour. But prior to all that, he'd say, "start the conversation." Stimp's advice would be to look up a Death Café (also known as "Café Mortale") in your area. These gatherings are a stellar beginning point, because they are *not* support groups—they merely provide space for folks to get together and talk about issues related to death (often having nothing to do with spirituality).

In his absence, Stimp's widow, Dr. Martha Taylor, continues to uphold Stimp's legacy as advocate for the dying and bereaved. Chatting with her continues to make me realize the *urgency* of having these conversations *now,* and helps me keep in mind the important things to consider—before it's too late.

In particular, as a dietician and professor, Martha has helped hospice staff, patients, and families with nutrition questions at the end of life. Her go-to advice for food at the end of life? "Let them eat *whatever* they want; feeding is such a part of feeling that we are nurturing and caring for our loved ones—it's part of comfort care. If they want juice or ice cream, let them eat it—they may even only want a taste of it." In keeping with her philosophy, Martha served ice cream at the reception following Stimp's memorial service. On that good advice, we gave Mom chocolate milkshakes in the hospital, *and* she enjoyed her favorite last meal: blueberry pancakes with nearly a gallon of syrup. And at mom's request, we served sweets at her memorial service.

Regarding more complex matters than food, in planning end-of-life care, *everyone,* Martha insists, should communicate with their chosen funeral home, crematorium, and/or hospice *far in advance* to see what services are available in their area.

Martha also taught me that, if one dies at home, there is no rush to have a body removed *immediately.* For families who wish to care for loved ones in a specific way (such as ritual prayer service or a bath after their loved one dies), or wish to simply sit with them, offering final goodbyes to the body of the person beloved in this life—this is totally appropriate. Our culture suggests that death is "bad" and our loved ones' bodies must be removed from the home as soon as possible following their deaths. This isn't necessarily the case. Of course, there are parameters and guidelines, but Martha encourages us to seek out wisdom from hospice, funeral homes, and crematoriums: "Ask professionals for whatever you need," including more time.

Lesson 2. Develop a Plan for Medical Events

Martha also suggests individuals connect with their local hospice on options in a *medical emergency.* For instance, if your loved one has a signed DNR and their M.O.S.T. papers, and does not wish to have *any curative care,* you do not necessarily need to call 9-1-1 if they have a medical event (e.g., stroke at home, heart attack, respiratory arrest, or cardiac arrest). You *can* phone hospice ahead of time to talk about options in case of a change in medical status.

For instance, if neither you nor your loved one want curative care at the end of life, and you (or they) have a stroke at home, are unable to speak or move, but are still conscious, it would be appropriate for hospice to take over their care if it's available in your area, as opposed to going to the emergency room for tests to be run. This is, of course, if you or your loved one have discussed this ahead of time, and would want to simply be made comfortable at home with palliative care. Your county or city's hospice can assist with talking through all these options ahead of time. So often, we *don't* think and plan ahead, and then, in the midst of a medical event, we become distressed and call 9-1-1, in lieu of connecting with hospice or putting our end-of-life care plan in motion.

If, as in our mom's case, your loved one is transported to a hospital and curative treatment begins—that's OK, but know that it is also OK to advocate for your loved one in the next steps. For us, it was "no surgery" for Mom. From conversations with Martha and Stimp—and my mom—I knew I needed to be fervent and aggressive, to attend to the legal paperwork, and to continue to advocate for my mom. Hospital doctors and surgeons are trained to fix medical problems, so you must make it clear if you or your loved one wish for comfort care instead.

Lesson 3: Honor Important Days and Honor Your Grief

It's been over two years since Stimp died, and his legacy lives on. Martha has taken care to grieve in her own way, including honoring important days with rituals that she and Stimp shared together. On the first anniversary of his death, she visited a retreat center they had attended together. She spent the day walking the grounds and the labyrinth. It helped her honor her own grief and remember his legacy. She continues to honor him and honor her own grief via Stimp's wisdom. In doing so, his name is lifted often, and his legacy of "starting the conversation" lives on. He would be proud.

Resource 7

Anticipating, Acknowledging, and Grieving Your Loss

Anticipated Grief: Love Letters and Bedside Conversations

A month before my mom's best friend died in September 2012 in inpatient hospice, I wrote her a letter. It was clear that the end was near, and her death was fast approaching. The grief was heavy; my anticipated loss of "Mama Phyllis" (my second mother) was overwhelming. I wanted to express to her how much I appreciated *all she'd done for me my entire life,* and how much I loved her and would always remember her. But I wasn't certain how to do it.

When a loved one's looming death is certain, and yet there is still time and you feel as if you have a lot left to say to them, letters work very well, especially when we feel bashful about telling our loved ones face-to-face how much they mean to us. Letters can also be useful if we feel we won't be able to say what we need to say when the time comes. That said, person-to-person or phone call conversations are deeply appreciated, too. Ron, Fred, and I had many a bedside conversation with Mom in hospice. We also encouraged her two siblings to phone her, since they could not be there in person. That worked exceptionally well, as Mom recognized and was very soothed by their voices.

As loved ones begin their journey toward death, it's imperative to keep all bedside conversations brief. This was a hard lesson for me, as the anticipated grief was monumental. I had so much I wanted to say to Mom. But dying loved ones do not have the energy for prolonged conversation. Simple reflections on gratitude, love, forgiveness, fond memories, legacy, and reassurance are useful. Above all, *presence* (being attentive—whether in person or via phone) is essential.

Acknowledging and Grieving Your Loss

Grief is a natural part of being in deep relationship and connection with others. Grief honors the threads of intimacy that weave us together as humans. Here are some steps in processing the grief.

Step 1: *Acknowledge the loss.* It took me years to acknowledge—aloud—that I had experienced a *lot* of loss. I hadn't realized the impact being the death chaplain had had on me, as well as the deaths of so many relatives, followed by Mom's. My work as a chaplain informed the ways in which I grieved all significant losses—including my parents. I had the tendency to go into "chaplain mode," which meant helping, doing, caregiving, and providing crisis management—rather than seeing myself as the one who *needed the help.* Because I was busy acting on others' behalf or holding *their* loss, I didn't do much with my own. It wasn't until after Mom died that I acknowledged that I had, indeed, suffered a significant, life-changing loss.

Step 2: *Acknowledge that grief comes in waves.* Grieving is not linear, though it can be cumulative. It's often triggered in unexpected ways—ordinary objects, memories, traffic intersections, songs, photos. When it arrives, grief can *feel* like an enormous wave crashing over us. It often feels as if it might swallow us whole amid a sea that *feels* fiercer than our ability to cope. Acknowledge these waves when they arrive, but know that they are not rip tides. They will not pull us into an ocean from which we cannot escape. We will not drown; we will not be lost at sea. We merely have to ride them out as they make their journey to shore.

Step 3: *Stay in the grief; don't minimize the loss; seek support.* Since grief *is* overwhelming, it can *feel* as if we are going to drown. Seek support—both professional and in close friends or family—to learn how to breath, tread water, float, and even paddle through the waves.

Chaplains, clergy, and hospice staff are all excellent resources to help you in navigating grief and adopting meaningful rituals on your journey. No two grief trains are alike; if you don't like a ritual, don't do it. If you like one ritual and want to do it repeatedly—do it. There are no rules. This is *your* grief train. The next section provides some suggestions—feel free to pass them along to loved ones currently grieving, and who may, ultimately, grieve *your* death.

Rituals for the Bereaved Following a Death

Following a loved one's death, grief can be a tough "train to ride." The following rituals are ways to help you cope with the loss. They can be adapted in any way you or your loved ones choose.

- Write a letter to your deceased loved one.

- Keep a grief notebook in which you write notes to your loved one, have a "conversation" with them, and jot down any feelings or experiences you have on your "grief train."

- Light a candle in remembrance. This could be done every day, on especially hard days, or on special occasions (birthdays, wedding anniversaries, anniversaries of death). In Judaism, these are called *yahrzeit* candles, and are typically lit on the anniversary of a death; they are designed to burn for 24 hours (For more information, visit Shiva.com.)

- Plant a tree, flower, or special plant in your loved one's honor.

- Make a blanket/quilt out of your loved one's favorite t-shirts or sweaters. If you do not sew, ask a local sewing shop whom they'd recommend to help you.

- Complete a service in honor of your loved one: volunteer for a nonprofit organization they liked, or engage in a community project they felt passionate about.

- Donate to your loved one's favorite charity.

- Commit random acts of kindness in your loved one's honor. A grieving friend of mine was once given $100 in $1 bills and told to share each of the bills in ways that would honor her deceased father. It gave her such a thrill to give away the money. She left bills on shelves in stores, left them in books, purchased others' orders for them, and donated in her father's name. Each time she used a bill, she felt her father's presence with her.

- Cook or eat your loved one's favorite food on special occasions (their birthday, holidays, anniversaries). As I've mentioned, my mother *loved* dessert—especially *chocolate*—so we always eat that in honor of her on special occasions.

- Do something special that your loved one enjoyed doing—or keep a ritual or tradition your loved one enjoyed. This could be during holidays, or could be as simple as a weekly or monthly ritual they did. *For example:* my mother loved Bob Evans restaurant and eating breakfast for any meal of the day. On television, she watched tennis obsessively (she was a Billy Jean King fan); liberal news channels, *Blue Bloods,* and *The Young and the Restless.* She enjoyed attending Durham Bulls baseball games each May, and she loved to pick up shells on the beach. Doing those things, now, connects me to her in a meaningful way.

- Reminisce over old photos and tell stories of the memories and people captured in the pictures. Organize your favorites into albums and share with loved ones. Recall the stories behind the photos.

- Hold a moment of silence or recite a special prayer or poem during family gatherings such as meals or reunions. Do the same if you are planning to scatter your loved one's ashes in a certain place. (We had this moment for Mom on the beach.)

- Keep their cherished photos or possessions out where you can see them each day—if it's not too painful. I keep photos of my mother and father on my dresser—and say, "Good morning," and, "Good night," to them each day.

- Tell stories and share fond memories of your loved ones. Do not be afraid to discuss and remember them. Lifting their names—at the dinner table, in everyday conversation—honors their legacy and acknowledges how much they are missed.

Theological Views of the Afterlife

In my own experience as a chaplain, professor, and grieving person, I realized that almost everyone facing loss looks at the "great chasm" and asks, "Will I see my loved one again?" Complex theological wonderings can arise from this simple inquiry, even if unanticipated. When this happens, we may turn to our religious and spiritual leaders, sacred texts, doctrine, and dogma for explanations. Know, however, that those tools may or may not provide *all* the answers—and that, even if they seem to, these may not be answers that necessarily satisfy you. And it's OK to *not* have all the answers. It's OK to be unsure of what, precisely, happens next. You are not alone. This is the nature of humanity.

The following are brief summaries of various afterlife theologies and rituals from the world's religious traditions that are offered here to provide some background. These are *not* exhaustive by any means. They merely provide a starting point for further inquiry and reading. (See the bibliography at the conclusion of this section.)

Christianity: Say Hello to Heaven

Christianity believes that life extends beyond our human, bodily "shells." This includes our eternal life in heaven or hell, or—in the Catholic tradition—our temporary life in purgatory. Heaven, in its broadest sense, is being in the eternal presence of God—whether that is a physical place, or merely a spiritual state of being. In Luke 23:43, Jesus describes heaven as "paradise," a place he will prepare for his followers. (See also Jn. 14:2–3).

Throughout the Christian teaching, heaven is also associated with a celestial place in which our physical bodies attain perfection and are made whole by the resurrection of the dead during Christ's second coming (1 Cor. 15; Phil. 3:20). This is why many Christians oppose cremation, for fear they will not experience bodily resurrection during that time.

Some view the afterlife as a physical heaven, where we may have physically perfected bodies. Others view heaven as simply a state of being. This idea comes from influence of Greek thought on Christianity—that the soul exists apart and outside of the body (duality) and time as we know it on earth (Brood et al 429). For Catholics, there is another aspect, a pit stop prior to heaven: purgatory. This is the space where souls endure temporary "refinement" to complete the work of reparation for sins committed on earth.

Orthodox Christianity, the earliest branch of the Christian church, teaches that souls enter a period of waiting after death, in which they can benefit from the prayers of their living loved ones (Brood et al 429). And Orthodox Christians will pray for loved ones' souls at various stages (days) after their deaths.

Hells Bells

Hell, like heaven, is another theological subject upon which Christians have not reached consensus (Grenz et al 37). Some Christians believe hell to be an actual place, while others espouse it to be a state of being in which the soul is eternally separated from God.

Brass Tacks: A Broad View of Christian Afterlife

Overall, the broad strokes view of Christianity's "Ultimate Purpose" is that the goal of life after death is for the soul to be in the presence of God for eternity.

Questions

Many questions about Christianity and the afterlife remain. Do we have our bodies in heaven—the place—or do our souls float about as we await Christ's second coming and our bodily resurrection? Or, are our souls merely *in* that eternal state of being called heaven? Is purgatory real? Is hell real? When it comes to Christian theology of the afterlife, there are more questions than answers.

Christianity and Reincarnation

When Fred and I wrestled over our fathers' fates, I began researching to see if there were any historical views in Christianity on reincarnation. In early Christianity, reincarnation was not completely off the table. Scripture alludes to this possibility in the story of the blind man's sin (see Jn. 9:2), as well as the question of John the Baptist's connection with Elijah (see Mt. 11:7–14) (Moreman 62). In the early formation of Christian doctrine and theology, reincarnation was prominent in the writing of early Church scholar Origen, as well as in gnostic theology, which considered the pre-existence of souls (Moreman 62 and Bache 150). But don't get too excited; *both* these were ruled as heretical—though individual Christians haven't abandoned the possibility of reincarnation completely.

Christopher M. Bache, professor of Religious Studies at Youngstown State University, for one, doesn't believe reincarnation to be incompatible with Christian theology. He writes, "Reincarnation represents an important link missing in Western theology" (Bache 151).

Again and Again: Hindu Teaching and the Afterlife

Hindu theology of the afterlife hinges on four theological concepts: the *atma, karma, samsara,* and *moksha.* An individual soul (*atma*) exists independently of the body or mind (and time and space for that matter). Somewhat like Christianity, the soul is eternal, but the key difference is that the soul has no beginning. It was never created and will never die. Just as God has no beginning or end, nor does God's energy, and the soul is one of those energies. The soul is always fully dependent upon its Source. Over unlimited lifetimes and endowed with varying degrees of free will, individual souls have blindly pursued ephemeral, sensual desires, causing them to harm other people, animals, or nature. The consequences of pursuing material and bodily desires are called *karma. Karma*—cause and effect—keeps the soul in a cycle of birth and death called *samsara,* which determines a soul's next birth. Liberation (*moksha)* from this cycle can only be obtained once mundane desires and *karma* have been fully and finally eliminated.

In Hinduism, God has unlimited forms that all correspond to a type of love that souls cultivate toward God. The goal of the spiritual practitioner is to serve and love God in aesthetic bliss (*rasananda*), similar to what Christianity would view as heaven.

Eliminating Desire: Buddhist Understandings of the Afterlife

Birthed out of Hinduism, Buddhism has a similar theological framework. The one large distinction is that most Buddhists do not worship nor believe in God or a deity. In Buddhism, the mind is propelled forward into the next birth based on its *karma* and desires, and *nirvana* is the ultimate purpose. The Buddha was not specific in his description of what *nirvana* looks or feels like—only that suffering ends with blowing out the flame of desire, and that allows the mind to be released from its endless cycle of life and death (Brood et al 184; Moreman 122, 123).

Anything Can Happen: Jewish Theology of the Afterlife

Judaism, with its diversity, embraces various theologies of the afterlife. Jewish scripture has little to say regarding the afterlife, and what happens after death is interpreted in various ways by various Jews on an individual level (Moreman 47). The concept of reincarnation is widespread in Judaism—particularly in Hasidism—as is the bodily resurrection (Moreman 151).

Unlike Christianity, Judaism does not believe the soul must be "saved" from its sin to reach its ultimate purpose. In Judaism, the High Holy Days, such as *Yom Kippur,* and weekly practices, such as *shabbat,* help humans progress morally and ethically both as individuals and as a community. Most Jews believe that the soul is immortal, but many disagree on what precisely happens to the soul at death (Brood et al 405). Many Jews place more of an emphasis on the world here and now, and *tikkun olam*: repairing the world through service and good works so that the Messiah will come.

Heaven Bound: Islamic Theology of the Afterlife

The majority of Muslims read the *Qur'an* (Islamic scripture) and understand the "Ultimate Purpose" in much the same way as Judaism and Christianity do (Moreman 74). Muslims believe that those who have followed the Five Pillars and lived righteously will enter paradise, and those who have lived unrighteous lives will be cast into hell (Brood et al 521).

Muslims also believe in the connection to the body after death, and its resurrection at the Judgement Day. The Qur'an affirms this belief: "Will He not cause you to die and restore you to life?" (Moreman 77). As in Judaism, proper burial of the dead is emphasized in Islam (Moreman 80).

The dominant question in Islam—very similar to Christianity—is the soul's timeline after death. Do souls travel immediately to heaven for a taste of eternity and then to their place of rest, to be bodily resurrected again, or do they remain in the grave until the Day of Judgement (Moreman 81, 85)? Or, does the soul go through a temporary place of refinement (like purgatory) in preparation for Judgement Day (Moreman 85)?

Bibliography for "Resource 8," and for Further Reading

- Bache, Christopher M. *Lifecycles: Reincarnation and the Web of Life*. Paragon House, New York, 1990.

- Brood, Jeffery, Layne Little, Brad Nystrom, Robert Platzner, Richard Shek, Erin Stiles. *Invitation to World Religions, Second Edition*. Oxford University Press, New York, 2015.

- Grenz, Stanley J., David Guretzki and Cherith Fee Nordling. *Pocket Dictionary of Theological Terms*. InterVarsity Press, Downers Grove, Ill., 1999.

- Moreman, Christopher. *Beyond the Threshold: Afterlife Beliefs and Experiences in World Religions, Second Edition*. Rowman and Littlefield, Lanham, Md., 2018.

Quotes and Scripture Passages about Death and Loss

"The Way It Is"
There's a thread you follow. It goes among
things that change. But it doesn't change.
People wonder about what you are pursuing.
You have to explain about the thread.
But it is hard for others to see.
While you hold it you can't get lost.
Tragedies happen; people get hurt
or die; and you suffer and get old.
Nothing you do can stop time's unfolding.
You don't ever let go of the thread.
—William Stafford

"She Is Gone"
You can shed tears that she is gone
or you can smile because she has lived.

You can close your eyes and pray that she will come back
or you can open your eyes and see all she has left.

Your heart can be empty because you can't see her
or you can be full of the love you shared.

You can turn your back on tomorrow and live yesterday
or you can be happy for tomorrow because of yesterday.

You can remember her and only that she's gone
or you can cherish her memory and let it live on.

You can cry and close your mind,
be empty and turn your back

or you can do what she would want:
smile, open your eyes, love and go on.
—David Harkins

Perhaps he knew, as I did not, that the Earth was made round so that we would not see too far down the road.
—Isak Dinesen, *Out of Africa*

"Sometimes" (excerpt)
Death waits for me, I know it, around
one corner or another.
This doesn't amuse me.
Neither does it frighten me.
—Mary Oliver

[D]o not fear, for I am with you,
do not be afraid, for I am your God;
I will strengthen you, I will help you,
    I will uphold you with my victorious right hand.
—Isaiah 41:10

"Do not let your hearts be troubled. Believe in God, believe also in me. In my Father's house there are many dwelling places. If it were not so, would I have told you that I go to prepare a place for you?"
—John 14:1–2

O death, where is thy sting? O grave, where is thy victory? The sting of death is sin; and the strength of sin is the law. But thanks be to God, which giveth us the victory through our Lord Jesus Christ.
—1 Corinthians 15:55–57 (KJV)

For now we see in a mirror, dimly, but then we will see face to face. Now I know only in part; then I will know fully, even as I have been fully known.
—1 Corinthians 13:12 (NRSV)

Indivisible, unburnable, insoluble,
all-pervading, changeless, unmoving, primeval,
invisible, inconceivable, and unchangeable, is the soul.
With this in mind, you should not mourn for the body.
—*Bhagavad-gītā* 2.24–25

For one who has been born, death is certain. For one who dies, a new birth is certain.
Therefore, do not lament the unavoidable.
—*Bhagavad-gītā* 2.27

Old clothes are discarded for new clothes.
In the same way, the soul discards old bodies for new ones.
—*Bhagavad-gītā* 2.22

At the end of life, remembering [God] while relinquishing the body, such a person attains [God], there is no doubt.
—*Bhagavad-gītā* 8.5

Notes and Further Reading

We're All Terminal: An Introduction to This Book

"We're all terminal... Some of us just have more information."
Kate Bowler, "My Prosperity Gospel," Festival of Faith and Writing Lecture, Friday, April 13, 2018, Grand Rapids Michigan.

Chapter 2: The Gas Will Be Gone Soon

Frank—a priest comforting author Kate Bowler after her Stage IV cancer diagnosis—had offered. "Don't skip to the end," he'd said.

Kate Bowler, *Everything Happens for a Reason: And Other Lies I've Loved* (New York: Random House, 2018), 160.

Chapter 5: Say Hello to Heaven

"What script are we using?" she said, "Which tab? Religious? Spiritual but not religious? Hope? Absurdity? Magical thinking? What is the meta-narrative, and what vocabulary list is most helpful?" Continuing, she also cautioned me to remember, "And so many times, the script flips."
Interview with Rev. Sally G. Bates, July 2018.

Chapter 6: Let's Talk about Death

"Ever since the diagnosis," she writes, "there has been a moment, in the minute between sleeping and waking, when I forget, when I have only a lingering sense that there is something I am supposed to remember."

Kate Bowler, *Everything Happens for a Reason: And Other Lies I've Loved* (New York: Random House, 2018), 66.

"I used to think that grief was about looking backward," Bowler writes. "I see now that it is about eyes squinting through tears into an unbearable future."

Kate Bowler, *Everything Happens for a Reason: And Other Lies I've Loved* (New York: Random House, 2018), 70.

From Didion I learned that "grief turns out to be a place none of us know until we reach it."

Joan Didion, *The Year of Magical Thinking* (London: Harper Perennial, 2006), 188.

"We can make some generalizations, certainly, about the train ride: shock and the five stages Elisabeth Kübler-Ross so famously outlines in her book, On Death and Dying. But the day-to-day grip of filling the void eludes us."

Joan Didion, *The Year of Magical Thinking* (London: Harper Perennial, 2006), 189.

"Only the survivors of death are truly left alone," Didion concludes. "The connections that made up their life...have all vanished."

Joan Didion, *The Year of Magical Thinking* (London: Harper Perennial, 2006), 193–94.

"The way you got side-swiped," wrote Didion, "was by going back."

Joan Didion, *The Year of Magical Thinking* (London: Harper Perennial, 2006), 112.

"We've banished both birth and death from our households, bedrooms, and parlors," she said, "and sent it off to the sterile land of modern medicine."

Interview with Rev. Sally G. Bates, July 2018.

"I want to die *naturally*....I've had a great life. When it's my turn to go, I'm ready."

Stimp Hawkins interview with Frank Stasio, host of *The State of Things* on North Carolina Public Radio, https://www.wunc.org/post/greensboro-man-celebrates-life-plans-death.

"Unknowns bring fear," he responded, corroborating Stimp's experience. "Most people will avoid anything that brings them fear."

Interview with Rev. Brad Mitchell, July 2018.

"I hadn't met her expectations, so she had missed the fact that I had adequately grieved in other ways," Brad said. "We have to be careful not to project our own way of grieving onto others— it's a weight they do not wish to bear."

Interview with Rev. Brad Mitchell, July 2018.

Chapter 7: Beginning with the End in Mind

But ...2,712,630 people died just in 2015 in the United States, or around 7,400 people per day.

CDC National Vital Statistics Report, November 2017.

"She would have had to have been a *smoked* ham," Sally added, because she, like my mother, appreciated the absurdity of it all.

Interview with Rev. Sally G. Bates, July 2018.

"Urns, hand-crafted boxes, mantelpiece clocks and statuary, fine gemstone jewelry—you can literally get *anything*," she told me. When her friend died just a day after July 4, she added, "His family said, 'Well, we could have packed him in a firecracker and shot him into space.'"

Interview with Rev. Sally G. Bates, July 2018.

Chapter 8: Savoring Life While Preparing for Death

"I did not tell them how few of their words are needed, but how much their hands are wanted, a hand on my back as I tear up, a hand on my head for a soft prayer of healing. When I feel I'm fading away, these hands prop me up and make me new."

Kate Bowler, *Everything Happens for a Reason: And Other Lies I've Loved* (New York: Random House, 2018), 75.

"Those words continue to remind me...we do not need to be minimizers of pain, the teachers of life lessons, nor the 'solutions to the problem' people when it comes to suffering, death, and grief."

Kate Bowler, *Everything Happens for a Reason: And Other Lies I've Loved* (New York: Random House, 2018), 116–18.

Dessert First Practical and Spiritual Resources

Resource 6: Stimp ("The Death Pimp") and Martha's Lessons on Savoring Life While Preparing for Death

Significant material found in this resource section was drawn from an interview with Dr. Martha Taylor, July 2018.

"Rituals for the Bereaved Following a Death," adapted from Transitions Hospice of Wake County "Ways to Honor and Remember Your Loved One."

Resource 8: Theological Views of the Afterlife

Bache, Christopher M. *Lifecycles: Reincarnation and the Web of Life*. Paragon House, New York, 1990.

Brood, Jeffery, Layne Little, Brad Nystrom, Robert Platzner, Richard Shek, and Erin Stiles. *Invitation to World Religions, Second Edition*. Oxford University Press, New York, 2015.

Grenz, Stanley J., David Guretzki, and Cherith Fee Nordling. *Pocket Dictionary of Theological Terms*. Intervarsity Press, Downers Grove, Ill., 1999.

Moreman, Christopher. *Beyond the Threshold: Afterlife Beliefs and Experiences in World Religions, Second Edition*. Rowman and Littlefield, Lanham, Md., 2018.

Acknowledgments

I didn't know it then, but this book began in a windowless conference room when a hiring committee determined that I was competent (enough) to matriculate into a prestigious Clinical Pastoral Education residency program. I'm grateful for that committee (you know who you are) and the chance they took on me. During our 2006–07 residency year, my fellow chaplains, supervisors, patients, and their families taught me to reflect on my own suffering, and to hold space for others to do the same. Thank you.

The biggest thanks goes to Ron, who was both doctor and son exemplar to Mom, and is brother extraordinaire to me. He has *always* been there for us both. Fred and Penny: you two are the best spouses Ron and I could ever hope for. Thank you for sticking with us. Your patience, endless support, and care for Mom did not go unnoticed.

Brad Lyons, Deborah Arca, Gail Stobaugh, and the entire Chalice Press team saw this book's potential and the possibilities it held for helping readers cope with life's most certain milestone. Joanna Bradley read the earliest pages as a sounding board. Molly Beck's eagle eye proofreading was a boon to this project. Thank you all.

There are numerous clergy and professionals who provided their stories and expertise on pastoral care and grief for this book. Rev. Carol D. Estes, Rev. Sally G. Bates, and Rev. Brad Mitchell: you are loved and appreciated. Dr. Martha Taylor: thank you for allowing me to share Rev. Stimp "The Death Pimp" Hawkins's wisdom, so that it may live on in perpetuity.

Immeasurable gratitude is also owed to best friends and family who knew intuitively how to care for an already moody writer digging deeply into the trenches of death and grief. These include

Britainy Sholl, Erin Riggs, Kate Harris, Joanna Bradley, Carol Estes, Heather Sanderson, and Barbara Jessie-Black.

Thank you to my patients, their families, and the staff at the hospital: you won't remember me—but I will never forget you. Thank you for the *honor* of inviting me into your rooms and hearts, allowing me to be present and care for you in the most sacred moment of life.

Finally, I offer heartfelt gratitude to Susan Read, Terry Huneycutt, Binkley Baptist Church, and Transitions Hospice of Wake County, North Carolina, for their care of our mom in her death—and their care of me in my life after her death.